To Sandy - Thank you for your interest.
Please share anything you learn.
Rob

Praise For Wellness Uprising

Rob Pell's <u>Wellness Uprising</u> provides a collection of interesting discussions that intelligently challenges what many would consider conventional wisdom in healthcare. But, most people don't know the history of the term conventional wisdom. It was originally coined by the noted economist John Kenneth Galbraith in his book <u>Affluent Society</u> in 1958. According to Galbraith conventional wisdom is established if it is simple, convenient, comfortable and comforting - though not necessarily true. Galbraith also said, "We associate truth with convenience with what most closely accords with self-interest or personal well-being." People want to believe conventional wisdom because it is indeed so simple, convenient, comfortable and comforting", even if it may not be true. And, once conventional wisdom on any topic is accepted, it becomes difficult to prove otherwise.

The reality is that the US medical establishment has created a conventional wisdom that drug-oriented medicine is the best form of medicine. Yet, many of these drugs only make us feel better in the short-term with the risk of dependency or producing side effects worse than the condition being treated for or causing the condition itself to worsen. The substantial risks and

D1010006

rising costs associated with a drug oriented medical system are creating an opportunity for change.

Change is definitely coming. In fact, we are in the midst of this change as there has been a subtle revolution occurring in medicine and a new paradigm is emerging. A paradigm refers to a model used to explain events. As our understanding of the environment and human body evolves, new paradigms (explanations) are developed. For example, in physics the cause and effect views of Descartes and Newton were replaced by quantum mechanics, Einstein's theory of relativity, and the theoretical physics that takes into considerations the tremendous "interconnectedness" of the universe.

The new paradigm in medicine also focuses on the interconnectedness of body, mind, emotions, social factors, and the environment in determining the status of health within an individual. And, while the old paradigm viewed the body basically as a machine that can be fixed best with drugs and surgery, the new model emerging utilizes these measures secondary to natural, non-invasive, techniques to promote health and healing.

I believe that the evolving paradigm will incorporate the best of both conventional and what is currently labeled as "alternative" medicine. Just as we now view the conventional treatments in vogue at the beginning of the 19th century (e.g., mercury, bloodletting, purges, etc.) as being irrational, counter-productive, and, in many cases, harmful, so too will many of today's conventional treatments be judged in a similar light by the medical circles of tomorrow. On the flip-side, there are many conventional medical practices and drugs that are completely rational. In fact, it would be irrational not to take advantage of modern medicine when appropriate. That said, there is no question that the majority of health complaints patients see doctors for owe their origin to dietary and lifestyle factors. Trying to treat the symptoms with a drug (a biochemical band-aid) often fails to address the underlying cause and leads to side effects as a result. Clearly, a more rational and truthful approach to healthcare is needed.

It is my sincere hope that you – or someone you care about – will use the information provided in Wellness Uprising to achieve greater health and happiness. I also hope that each of you can become advocates of change. As Dr. Martin Luther King, Jr. said, "duration is not enough: the mere passage of time does not create change. It requires ordinary people envisioning, acting and constructing the future."

Live in good health with passion and joy!

Michael T. Murray, ND

As an Integrated Medical physician in Oregon for over 25 years I strive to guide and educate patients to a state of balance, wholeness, and health.

This process is accomplished through empowering them to take the initiative to create a lifestyle which will foster reintegration of body, mind, and spirit. Education and instruction are crucial elements of this process which makes it a delight to **enthusiastically endorse** Rob Pell's book, Wellness Uprising.

It's teeming with vital health-enhancing data that serves to not only inform but also to inspire. Mr. Pell masterfully shares his extensive knowledge in a no-nonsense yet humorous manner, empowering the reader to awaken from the hypnotic trance the Western medical model has them in. The book is highly readable, enjoyable and invaluable, taking on Big Pharma, Big Farming, and the government agencies that are supposed to oversee public health.

Many thanks to Rob for his wonderful contribution to our community and for all those he's inspired to reclaim their birthright of radiant health. Let Rob show you real health is a lot simpler than you've been led to believe!

I'm certain that <u>Wellness Uprising</u> will "fly off" my shelf, his shelf and many others as well.

Steven Rotter MD
Integrated Medical Physician
Grants Pass, Or.

WELLNESS UPRISING

Your Health In Your Hands

Dedication and Acknowledgments

Wellness Uprising is dedicated to the increasing number of Americans who have a strong sense that "something just ain't right" with the US healthcare system – even if they can't pinpoint exactly what it is. It is my belief that daily reliance on toxic drugs is, in most cases, very damaging to people's long-term well-being. It is my hope that this book will help them make the decision to avoid using toxic, drug-centered treatments for their primary healthcare – there is a much better way.

I would also like to acknowledge all of my teachers including my wife and our four children. In their different ways, they each helped make this book a reality.

A special thanks to my insightful editors, Tyler, Alysia, and Dan, who helped keep me focused and on track while encouraging me to take the time necessary to expand examples and explanations for greater clarity.

Rob Pell

"All truth passes through three stages. First, it is ridiculed. Second, it is violently opposed. Third, it is accepted as being self-evident."
– Arthur Schopenhauer

Published by:
Midnight Star Publishing
Grants Pass, Oregon

For more information, please contact the author directly:
Email: RobertPell9@gmail.com
Phone: 877.656.1634

ISBN: 0692261281
ISBN 13: 9780692261286

Table of Contents

Please note: As the author is not a licensed healthcare practitioner, nothing in this book should be considered a substitute for advice from your doctor. Before beginning or discontinuing any medical treatment, readers should always consult with their doctor.

Foreword

<u>Wellness Uprising</u> is a compelling book for our times. With increasing numbers of people suffering from chronic illnesses that are largely preventable, those seeking a healthier path need a guide that is both informative and practical to help them achieve and maintain the vibrant health that should be everyone's birthright.

Since becoming a physician in 1982, I have dedicated my career to helping people get healthy and stay healthy using natural, non-toxic methods. Early in my training I saw that conventional means for treating chronic diseases did not work, and often led to complications and further problems. As a seeker and lover of the truth, I have always been keenly aware when I encountered a book that spoke the unvarnished truth. <u>Wellness Uprising</u> is such a book.

I have known Rob Pell for over 25 years. When I moved to Boston, MA, in the mid 80s, I was naturally drawn to The Five Seasons, the natural foods restaurant Rob and his two brothers owned and operated. Rob poured his heart, soul, and integrity ... and of course his considerable knowledge of good quality food and cooking ... into the restaurant. I know because I dined there at least once a week, often more, for many years. The food was always high quality, healthful, and great tasting; and Rob was almost always on site in the kitchen.

Rob's current venture, Sunshine Natural Foods, has provided him with another platform for providing great food, and beyond that, excellent and necessary health advice to his clients. The book you are holding represents the culmination of his many years of research and experience regarding all subjects natural and holistic.

Clearly Rob loves what he does and is very good at it. As you read this book you will see that he is a man who speaks his truth, no matter how nonconforming it is to the conventional "wisdom" of our times. You will also discover that he practices what he preaches when it comes to living a healthy lifestyle. His own vitality is evident throughout the book, and he encourages his readers to follow his example, take charge of their lives, and become their own health experts.

Included are chapters on several aspects of food and nutrition, exercise, sleep, stress management, alternatives to drugs, toxins to avoid (in cookware, water, cell phones, pet food, sunscreen and pharmaceuticals), and much more. Very important chapters on caring naturally for our most precious resource, our children, are featured. No matter how much you already know, you will know more after reading this book. It contains a wealth of information on numerous topics.

<u>Wellness Uprising</u> is a book that will inform you about why you need to live more healthfully, and gives you practical tools on how to do so. Perhaps more important, it will ignite the inspiration and passion within you to make the changes necessary to realize ongoing health and wellbeing.

Janet Levatin, MD
Holistic Pediatrician, Tenpenny Integrative Medical Center
Former Clinical Instructor in Pediatrics, Harvard Medical School

Introduction

One of my dreams is for people everywhere to empower themselves through holistic health education, so they can avoid being dependent on the pharmaceutical industry dominated drug delivery system for primary healthcare. That is the reason I wrote this book.

During a health crisis you don't need a PhD, but you will need to know as much about your own health and wellness as your doctor knows about drugs and disease. That way, even if you choose to visit a doctor, you will know enough to be able to ask him good questions. **Good questions should lead to better answers. Better answers should generate more confidence and more confidence will make it more likely his recommendations will be effective.** It can be win-win-win. Nonetheless, learning when it's appropriate to say "No" to your doctor can be a lifesaving skill.

Anyone who has been in my natural food store knows I often speak with authority about many health-related subjects. The ultimate source of my authority goes far beyond my individual studies, it's rooted in the real-world, personal health stories thousands of our customers generously share. I do my best not to jump to hasty conclusions. However, when I'm told dozens, hundreds, or sometimes thousands of very similar stories that effectively confirm each other, I'm comfortable repeating them so we can all benefit from each others' experiences. Ultimately, if a product in my store sits on the shelf collecting dust, it's either overpriced or it doesn't work. If a product flies off the shelf, month after month, year after year, the customers have spoken - loud and clear - the product works! The free-market often has a way of making things crystal clear.

"Universal Healthcare" usually refers to a system that provides healthcare and financial protection to all citizens. It is organized around providing a specified package of benefits to all members of a society with the end goal of providing financial risk protection, improved access to health services, and improved health outcomes.

In fact, using your body in the way it was designed is the best way to pay the "premium" for true, universal healthcare. Virtually all members of society have this option available. The pages of this book are dedicated to the thesis that every living organism on this planet had the ability to enjoy perfect health - long before Monsanto (GMOs), DuPont (better living through chemistry) or drug giants like AstraZeneca, Merck, Novartis, Pfizer, and others lobbied (paid) their way into the controls of government regulating agencies like the Food and Drug Administration (FDA) and the Environmental Protection Agency (EPA).

The chapters of this book will in many cases provide the information you need to make good health decisions. In other cases, it may help you to ask your doctor better questions. I believe the title of the first chapter says a lot: *The "Latest" Health Secrets Have Been Around For Thousands Of Years.* Taking careful note of what health and wellness strategies have proven succesful for centuries, can help you become your own health expert.

Thousands of our customers say that my newspaper health columns and store newsletters help them make better, easier, more informed health decisions. Unbiased, accurate health information can make our lives easier.

In the first decade of raising our four children, my wife and I made only three trips to an MD for help with the kids. The first time was when one young daughter got into my wife's sewing supplies and managed to get a small button caught in her ear. We couldn't get it out and went to the doctor to remove it. The second time, another daughter got an uncooked navy bean caught up her nose and we went again for help with removal. The last visit was to the same doctor to remove a large, painful splinter. We used no drugs, no hospital delivery rooms, no well baby visits, no vaccines, no antibiotics, and had nearly no medical expenses. In the next 16 years, before our youngest left the nest, we visited MDs with the kids only two more times. Those were for X-rays and treatment of relatively minor sports injuries.

Common sense (maybe not so common anymore), honest effort, some smarts, and a little luck were enough to raise a healthy family.

Rob Pell

1

The "Latest" Health Secrets Have Been Around For Thousands Of Years

Beware Of Big Pharma's Patented "Improvements" to Nature

In the information-obsessed culture we live in, people have been conditioned to believe that "new" automatically equates to better. While books, magazines, newspapers, and medical schools focus obsessively on the latest health research, **I've never been able to figure out: what's wrong with the oldest health research?**

Some new medical technologies are absolutely amazing. Replacement knees and hips can provide decades of pain-free mobility to otherwise healthy people who want to continue living healthy active lifestyles. But many others, like the multitude of drugs advertised during the nightly news, have such a long, almost laughable, list of possible side effects, "including death," that sane people have to wonder if there is not a better approach to wellness.

1

Perfect, drug-free health every day is the birthright of all living things, rich and poor, young and old ... all of us. If you're not sure if a health or dietary practice makes sense, ask yourself these simple questions: has it withstood the test of time? Not just thirty or forty years, but has it worked well for three or four hundred years, or more? Is it truly healthy and natural? Or, is it just another profit-driven fad - a quick-fix being marketed as the next great breakthrough? Far too often we see health "breakthroughs" from 10 years ago become health nightmares 10 years from now. The list of tragic drug recalls grows every year; and remember that every drug that has ever been recalled was at one time given a "seal of approval" by the Food and Drug Administration (FDA). Only methods that are time-tested to be truly safe and that really work become long-lasting traditions.

As you read this book please remember: vibrant, drug-free health is the real normal (don't let pharmaceutical company ads convince you otherwise). By being proactive and working together sharing accurate information, we can all help chart the course of a Wellness Uprising!

The "New Normal"

The list of what is becoming the **"new normal"** for health in America is amazing and disturbing. An average of over 13 drug prescriptions are now written annually for every man, woman, and child in the country with one in ten Americans using prescription antidepressants. American Academy of Pediatrics recommendations now state that children should receive 35 vaccine doses by the age of 15 months, 49 doses by age six, and 69 doses by age 18! Public health officials in New York City recently declared a "diabetes epidemic." Cases of type 2 diabetes have increased 90% in the last decade and childhood diabetes is being called the *new epidemic* in American kids.

In children, soaring autism rates, serious ADHD issues, life-threatening acute allergies, and asthma are all becoming part of the "new normal" childhood. Anaphylactic shock produced by peanut exposure has caused many schools across the country to ban peanut butter sandwiches (the public school my grandson attends features *peanut-free zones*). Inhalers in kids' backpacks and lunch boxes are now commonplace. All 50 states have laws allowing students to carry and self-administer these medications during their school day. The Centers for Disease Control (CDC) and The American Lung Association acknowledge this but offer no reasonable explanations.

Dr. Grant Tomkinson, of the University of South Australia, examined 50 studies on running fitness that involved more than 25 million children from 28 countries. He stated, **"In the one mile run, the typical child of today would finish about one and a half minutes behind the typical child of 1975."**

Old Normal

Growing up in the 60s, I cannot recall anyone who was prevented by asthma from running around all day long with the rest of us, or was allergic to peanut butter, or had even heard of type 2 diabetes in children. The most common anti-depressant drug, Prozac, hadn't even been invented. **That's probably because *real* normal was, is, and always will be - being healthy, active, and drug free every day.**

3

Battle Between The Two "Normals"

We are now witnessing and experiencing a high-stakes battle between the two normals. One dictionary definition of "War" is, *a struggle or competition between opposing forces* (or ideas) *for a particular end*. By that definition, this is a war and the particular end being fiercely contested is control of our core beliefs about health. The stakes are high both in dollars and quality of life, and in some cases unintended death.

On one side of the battle lines align forces trying to convince us that we can all adapt comfortably to our "new normal" world by simply using enough patented pharmaceuticals. Most medical doctors must be entrenched in this camp because over four billion prescriptions for drugs are now written annually in the US. According to IMS Institute for Healthcare Information, prescription drug sales in the US now exceed $340 billion annually. A York University (Toronto Canada) study, concluded that **nearly twice as much is spent by the US pharmaceutical industry on drug advertising and promotion than is spent on actual research.** In some cases it seems that even government watchdog agencies that are supposed to protect us, like the FDA, align with the pharmaceutical companies in the quest to convince us that their products are an indispensable part of *new normal* daily life.

People on the other side believe or understand that in times of sickness, your body does everything possible to heal and repair itself – to re-establish your normal healthy condition – and usually succeeds with no medical intervention at all if provided with basic wellness supporting building-blocks. Virtually all naturopathic doctors (ND), chiropractors, acupuncturists, Integrative Medicine practitioners, and some forward-thinking MDs are in this camp.

Control over the strategic decision-making 'territory' between our ears has become just as important to pharmaceutical corporate giants (Big Pharma) as production site, pipeline, and trade route control is to oil producing corporate giants. **Command of information flowing into that sensitive region (your brain) is directly tied to Big Pharma's bottom line profits.**

Irrespective of the happy images that carefully choreographed pharmaceutical company ads portray of people using their drugs, there is no getting around the fact that staying truly healthy and in balance requires using our bodies at least somewhat within the parameters of the way that they were designed. Clean food grown from rich soil, clean (non-chlorinated) water, some regular moderate physical activity, and natural (drug-free) sleep, are now and have always been, the non-negotiable, true building-blocks of a healthy life.

The Time-Tested, Four Pillars Of Health

1) Good Food

People can thrive eating many types of healthy diets. Some choose to rely on animal-based sources of concentrated protein and fats while others choose vegetarian sources - either can work well. Regardless of whether you are an omnivore or observe one of the different types of vegetarian diets, eating moderate amounts of whole unprocessed organic food is a primary component of a healthy lifestyle. Ironically, until the last one or two hundred years, it's the only diet that was even available.

Eating vegetables is *very* important. Whatever diet you choose, I would recommend that it include at least 50% to 60% vegetables, with most of them being of the green-leafy variety.

Choosing foods that are grown and produced using well established organic methods is paramount. If a farming practice has been productive for a thousand years, it will continue to be passed on. If a farming practice didn't work a thousand years ago, the village starved and the practice was abandoned - simple. Modern chemically dependent farming methods, especially those featuring genetically modified organisms (GMOs) and the extra Roundup herbicide that goes with them, are *far from proven*. In fact, in the US there have been no long or medium-term safety tests, done by the FDA or the Environmental Protection Agency (EPA), on GMOs at all.

Every living organism on the planet (with the notable exception of modern man and his pets), naturally eats what grows, or can be stored easily, in its immediate ecosystem. This creates balance with the environment. Balance results in health, imbalance in disease. Wild animals and plants in a balanced, natural setting seldom, if ever, get sick. This is as true today as it was a thousand years ago.

Regularly consuming large quantities of refined sugars is definitely one part of the "new normal" American diet that you would be smart to avoid. The US diet has changed dramatically in the last 200 years. In 1822, an average American consumed 6.3 lbs. of refined sugar per year. The average American now consumes over 100 lbs. of refined sugar per year. Obesity researcher Stephan Guyenet described it another way: In 1822, the average American consumed, over the course of about a week, the same amount of sugar found in one of today's 12 ounce soft drinks. Now, we consume that much every 7 hours. This is a very unhealthy trend and clearly an example of *new* not being better. It is one of the obvious factors contributing to the skyrocketing obesity and diabetes rates in the US.

2) Moderate Exercise

From TV fixation to hours at the computer or years on a job that only exercises our hands and brains, many of us live unnatural sedentary lifestyles. Americans' most popular "activities" which includes driving, are done while sitting. But that is not what we were designed for.

A simple half hour walk, three or more days a week, has a myriad of well documented physical and emotional health benefits. It's proven that regularly taking a brisk walk especially in fresh air is good for the heart, reduces cholesterol and blood sugar, improves mood, reduces stress, improves sleep, clears the mind and strengthens bones. If humans were given an "owners manual" at birth, walking would probably be included for routine maintenance of every body system. No fancy spandex or gym memberships needed for a walk, just a good pair of shoes and enough will power to put one foot in front of the other.

Walking is probably the simplest and least expensive (usually free) form of regular exercise and it is only one example. To increase your chances of staying motivated to exercise you should choose activities you enjoy doing that also elevate your heart rate, and make sure to do them at least three or more times per week.

3) Pure Water

No living creature on the planet ever naturally consumes chlorinated water. Chlorine is a necessary evil for municipalities to supply microbe-free water to our homes. However, filtering out the chlorine before use is the only practice that makes sense. In his book, <u>Coronaries Cholesterol Chlorine</u>, Dr. Joseph

Price demonstrates the link between ingesting chlorinated water and increased risk of cardiovascular disease. Chlorinated water has also been conclusively shown to increase risk of bladder and colon cancers. A simple chlorine-removing filter will cost you pennies a gallon. People drinking their own well water are usually fine.

Drink enough pure water to keep from ever being thirsty for very long. While obvious in summer, during winter, wood or forced-air heat can be very drying and needs to be considered.

4) Deep Sleep

For thousands of years, humans naturally allowed the sun and the seasons to determine their sleep-wake cycle. Man is not naturally a nocturnal animal. Each day, when darkness arrives and the temperature drops, your body's pineal gland begins to secrete melatonin, the sleep hormone. Within a few hours, sleep should naturally follow. This natural health promoting cycle is disrupted by artificial lights, late-night TV-watching, and computer use. Your circadian rhythm (or sleep-wake cycle) drives the rhythms of biological activity throughout your body at the cellular level. Negative effects from sleep disruptions affect all body systems.

Dr. Charles Czeisler, head of the Division of Sleep Medicine at Harvard Medical School said, "sleep is the third pillar of health." Sleeping for seven to eight hours a night has been proven to positively impact blood pressure, memory, immunity, mental health, obesity, longevity, and much more, compared with sleeping less than six hours a night. Further, sleeping for seven to eight hours a night has been linked to positive personality characteristics such as optimism and greater self-esteem.

Health Bonus For Humans

Humans are one of the only animals who have the ability to appreciate humor. Laughter has proven to boost immunity, increase your body's natural feel-good chemicals, and is fun and free! Remember to find reasons to laugh. You're never too old (or young) to laugh, exercise, eat and drink healthily.

Using your body in the way it was designed is the best way to pay the "premium" for true, universal healthcare. The odds of fully healing, repairing and being completely healthy, go way up when you provide your body with the time-tested four healthy basics. During a health crisis you don't need a PhD, but you will need to know as much about your own health and wellness as your doctor knows about drugs and disease.

2

The Nation's #1 Killer
Is Easily Avoided

*Learning To Say "No" To Your Doctor
Can Be A Life-Saving Skill*

In recent years, the discussion over unnecessary and preventable deaths has reached a fever pitch. Where shall we begin? In the United States annual gun related homicides total about 11,000, automobile fatalities are about 35,000 per year, and close to 20,000 people die each year because of sexually transmitted diseases (STDs).

Would you be surprised to learn that the leading cause of preventable death in the US is the medical system itself? This is the startling conclusion reached in the comprehensive and meticulously documented report titled *Death By Medicine* published by medical researchers: Gary Null, PhD; Carolyn Dean MD, ND; Martin Feldman, MD; Debora Rasio, MD; and Dorothy Smith, PhD.

Deaths resulting from inadvertent, adverse effects or complications from medical treatment or diagnostic procedures are known as iatrogenisis, meaning: brought forth by a healer

11

(from the Greek *iatros*, healer). Their report places the number of annual iatrogenic deaths in the US at a staggering 783,936.

Hippocrates, the ancient Greek physician, is often regarded as the "Father of Western Medicine." Ninety-eight percent of American medical students swear to some form of the Hippocratic Oath before practicing medicine. One of the underlying principles of the Oath is: *"first, do no harm."* I'm not sure if that's sad or ironic.

Today, the largest contributors to iatrogenic deaths are prescription drugs being *used as directed.* According to a report issued by *Medical News Today*, over 4 billion prescriptions were written for drugs in America in 2011. That's an average of over 13 for each man, woman and child. The average number of prescriptions written annually for a senior citizen is 28 per year. That doesn't include over-the-counter medications or vaccines.

Some might consider doctors unsuspecting, even well-meaning pawns of Big Pharma. Non-apologists consider them street level pushers for FDA sanctioned drug cartels. Either way, the drug kingpins couldn't deliver the goods without MDs helping them complete their drug delivery cycle.

If these drugs could successfully treat and cure disease, the United States would have the healthiest inhabitants on the planet. In reality, there is no positive correlation between prescription medication and good health; in fact, the opposite is probably true.

The possible adverse reaction warnings on TV drug commercials make fantastic material for stand up comedians, but, life-threatening side-effects are no laughing matter. Common side-effects of individual drugs are well publicized but it's impossible for physicians and pharmacists to reliably predict what possible side-effects will occur when combining 3, 4, 13, or 28 different drugs.

I was recently saddened to read the obituary of one of my customers, a strongly-built US Navy veteran in his mid-seventies, who appeared to be fit and in excellent health a few years ago. He was found dead, lying on the floor of his residence. His sudden, unexplained death inspired me to write this chapter after his son told me he had reviewed his dad's prescriptions with him about a year ago and was shocked to discover that **seven of the twelve drugs his father was taking had been prescribed to treat side-effects from one of the other drugs. No autopsy was performed to determine the cause of death.**

The *Journal of the American Medical Association* (JAMA) published a study by Dr. Barbara Starfield, an MD with a Master's degree in Public Health, revealing the extremely poor performance of the United States healthcare system in terms of preventable death. One of Starfield's chief concerns is a lack of systematic recording and studying of adverse events stemming from prescription drugs. If a patient dies, there is no routine procedure to notify their physician, even if the patient is autopsied. **Therefore, there is almost no way for the average doctor to link a patient's death to a possible adverse reaction to a prescribed medication.**

This is especially troubling because another article published in JAMA concluded prescription drugs *used as directed* cause about 106,000 deaths a year and over two million serious injuries annually in the US. This makes prescription drugs the single largest factor in all non-natural deaths in our nation, and these deaths happen to be caused directly by the routine practices of the medical establishment. Astonishingly, this figure makes the combined death figure of homicide, auto collisions, and STDs pale by comparison.

Only about 20%, or one in every five deaths nationwide are subject to investigation by a coroner or medical examiner. If an attempt to find cause of death through an autopsy was mandatory, I'm certain that the number of deaths actually caused by prescription drugs, used as directed, would dwarf the 106,000 per year the JAMA report concluded.

Due to concerns about dangerous side-effects from long-term use, many prescription drugs were at one time specifically prescribed only for short-term use. Now just a few years later, many of the same drugs are routinely prescribed, indefinitely, for the rest of your life. Prescriptions for drugs are seldom written to enhance the patient's fundamental well-being but rather to simply shut off symptoms, which almost always makes them a poor choice for long-term use.

I've seen enough to convince me that corporate pharmaceutical giants like Pfizer, Merck, and AstraZeneca (Big Pharma), which are some of the largest corporations – period – are far more concerned with creating repeat, lifetime customers rather than with finding cures. But drug companies don't act alone. Along with those Pharmaceutical giants, the FDA and insurance companies have become kingpins of this profit-driven business model. Some might consider doctors unsuspecting, even well-meaning, pawns of Big Pharma. Non-apologists consider them street level pushers for FDA sanctioned drug cartels. Either way, the kingpins couldn't legally deliver the goods without medical doctors helping them complete the drug delivery system.

Dr. Robert Epstein, chief medical officer of Medco Health Solutions Inc. (a unit of Merck & Co.), oversees drug-benefit plans for more than 60 million Americans, including 6.3 million seniors who receive more than 160 million prescriptions. Conducting a study in 2003 of drug trends among the elderly, he found it common for seniors to see multiple physicians, get multiple prescriptions, and use multiple pharmacies. This makes it extremely difficult for physicians to get an accurate overview of a patient's total care.

> The number of antibiotics prescriptions written for viral infections is 20 million per year. Antibiotics have no effect on viruses, however. This practice of over prescribing is inexplicable and inexcusable.

Death by Medicine also reported that the number of people exposed to unnecessary hospitalization annually is 8.9 million per year. And the number of unnecessary medical and surgical procedures performed is 7.5 million per year. This is cause for concern because a 2008 study issued by the *Office of Inspector General for the Department of Health and Human Services*, reported that one in seven Medicare beneficiaries who is hospitalized will be harmed as a result of the medical care they receive in the hospital.

Prescription drugs and hospital visits are very risky business. Unlike with other more well-publicized causes of death, simply taking greater personal responsibility for our own health and well-being and learning how to say "No" to your doctor could save hundreds of thousands of lives every year. More gun or traffic laws or sex education classes will do nothing to save us from what is actually the nation's number one killer, the US medical system.

3

Healthy Alternatives To The Mainstream Medical System

The Seven Levels Of Healing

Many people believe that Western medicine is so advanced it should *always* be the first choice for all our healthcare needs. Actually, nothing could be further from the truth. There are definitely times when Western medicine is the best and most appropriate healthcare choice. In cases of acute trauma from a serious accident, there is no doubt that a modern emergency room and talented surgeons can save lives.

However for long-term care of a chronic condition, I believe you would enjoy better treatment from a doctor in China 1,000 years ago than you'd get from a Western doctor today. Virtually any long-term treatment (drugs) a Western doctor prescribes for a chronic condition will almost always have long-term, toxic side effects - which today's doctors may, or may not, fully understand. With over four billion prescriptions written annually in the US and the average American now receiving 13 prescriptions for drugs a year, poorly understood drug side-effects are a major cause for concern. Further, it is virtually impossible to predict with certainty the effects of simultaneously using several different drugs, which can make the use of prescription drugs a real roll of the dice.

In addition to toxic medications, in today's world exposure to environmental toxins in our air, water, and food supplies is almost unavoidable. The list of proven toxins is very long. It includes over 17,000 pesticides and herbicides alone, plus chlorine, plastics, fragrances (laundry and personal care products), PCBs in farmed fish, and a lot more. If bodily systems are preoccupied with neutralizing or clearing toxins, it leaves less energy for regeneration, and healing will be impaired. Doing everything reasonably possible to avoid toxic exposures is a very important step toward optimizing health. Most Western MDs seldom mention anything about this basic truth.

However, if you believe that the human birthright is to live a healthy life and that vibrant health is the normal condition for your body, you're halfway to achieving that goal. You already understand that in times of sickness your body does everything possible to heal and repair itself – to re-establish your normal healthy condition – usually with no medical intervention at all.

As a guide to knowing *where to shop* for healthcare I offer you my concept of ***The Seven Levels Of Healing***. Integrating this philosophy into your daily life, you'll find that the least costly treatment with the fewest side effects will usually provide the most long-term benefit. **The basic premise is that, beginning with level one, you always try the simplest, yet often the most profound, levels of healing before turning to more complex**

solutions at the bottom of the list. The higher the level (smaller number), the cost is typically lower, the effects more wide-ranging, and the side-effects fewer.

The Seven Levels Of Healing

⚮ **Level 1)** Intentional positive attitude shift and thought adjustment is sometimes all it takes to improve your health. This can be the strongest, most profound "medicine" of all. This may not sound measurable or scientific, but regularly visualizing change can often be the needed catalyst towards achieving it.

⚮ **Level 2)** Fresh air, relaxation and deep breathing - thereby increasing oxygen - decreasing stress and clearing the mind has been used for centuries. Absorbing fresh energy and gratitude (inspiration) when inhaling and releasing stress and negative baggage when exhaling, can be very effective in creating your own sense of lasting well-being. Recently scientists have figured out that this stuff really works. Some might call this meditation. Scientists call it relaxation response therapy.

⚮ **Level 3)** Dietary changes and improved eating habits make a huge difference. Cancer, heart disease, diabetes, and obesity can all be greatly affected by food choices. Astonishingly, it took the most esteemed doctor in the US, the Surgeon General, until 1988 to acknowledge the basic truth that food matters. To our grandmothers and probably all grandmothers in history, this truth was self-evident. Herbs and supplements would be included on this level.

⚮ **Level 4)** Energy based mind-body integration and rejuvenation exercises like the ancient practices of yoga, tai chi and chi gung can create lasting health improvements. Western forms of cardiovascular exercise may be included here if they are done with an emphasis of coordination, rhythm and pace, deep breathing, de-stressing, relaxing the mind, and rejuvenating the body. These could include: walking, jogging, swimming, and cross-country skiing.

⅄ **Level 5)** Massage, Chiropractic, Physical Therapy, and other forms of hands-on body-work serve to re-establish and adjust the alignments and relationships between the body's moving parts. They also help to reduce the effects of stress and overuse.

⅄ **Level 6)** Acupuncture has traditionally been used to reestablish energetic balance and to fully engage *all* your body's healing systems in a coordinated way. Although marginally invasive, the use of tiny acupuncture needles is usually completely painless. Modern medical electrical stimulation techniques take a small page out of acupuncture books and also work directly with the body's energy channels. Many athletic trainers now use electronic devices (instead of acupuncture needles) to manipulate the body's energy flows to bring athletes back to competition quicker. Over the years, my body has responded very well to traditional acupuncture.

⅄ **Level 7)** Drugs and surgery are costly, invasive and often dangerous. Plus, the long-term side-effects are often very scary or unknown. It would be wise to use them only after methods from the other 6 levels have been tried.

Notice that everything on levels one through six readily lend themselves to being complementary and synergistic. Actions and attitudes from these levels can often make actions from Level 7 more effective as well. Unfortunately, most MDs (often due to their lack of holistic health understanding) place Level 7 procedures alone on a pedestal. They routinely fail to integrate the simpler, less costly, complementary practices from the other levels as follow-up that could make their Level 7 treatments more effective and long lasting.

Dr. Andrew Weil is the world's most well-known Integrative Health practitioner, a Harvard trained MD, has appeared on the cover of Time Magazine twice, and was named one of the 100 most influential people in the world. In his groundbreaking, best-selling, book <u>Spontaneous Healing</u>, Weil wrote: **"When I finished my basic clinical training, I made a conscious decision not to practice the kind of medicine I had just learned.** I did so for two reasons, one emotional and one logical. The first was simply a gut feeling that if I were sick, I would not want to be treated the way I had been taught to treat others, unless there was no alternative. That made me uncomfortable. The logical reason was that most of the treatments I had learned in four years at Harvard Medical School and one of internship did not get to the root cause of disease processes and promote healing but rather suppressed those processes or merely counteracted the visible symptoms of the disease. **I had learned almost nothing about health and its maintenance, about how to prevent illness - a great omission, because I had always believed that the primary function of doctors should be to teach people how *not to get sick* in the first place.** The word "doctor" comes from the Latin word for "teacher." Teaching prevention should be primary; treatment of existing disease, secondary."

In the last forty years I have engaged the services of MDs for myself four times. In those instances, options from the top six levels were simply not enough to do the job. Those four visits could best be characterized as relatively minor repairs to injured body parts pushed beyond the limits of common sense. I used no prescription or over-the-counter drugs in the aftercare.

The circumstances for two of the instances were these: in the early nineties I was windsurfing in the strong winds of Oregon's Columbia River Gorge - traveling at about 30 mph when my board's fin hit a sandbar causing it to come to an instantaneous stop. Problem was, only the board stopped. I continued, flying forward at 30 mph, landing on my feet, 25 feet away, in ankle-deep water to the unmistakable popping sounds of unhappy cartilage in my knees. Both knees (years later at different times) eventually needed to have a small piece of damaged cartilage removed to prevent the joints from periodically locking up. In both cases, in the weeks following the minor surgeries, instead of pain meds (although they were certainly offered), I used ice, acupuncture, massage, and anti-inflammatory herbs and enzymes to hasten recovery. There are times when employing the services of a medical doctor is appropriate.

Why resort to complex, costly or dangerous solutions if simple and inexpensive approaches would work well? Why risk the toxic side effects of drugs that may be worse than the condition they were used for, if a daily half-hour walk might do the job? The levels on which you regularly "shop" for your healthcare will ultimately help determine your long-term well-being.

4

Organic Farming Is
The Only Smart Choice

Healthy Strong Crops Lead To
Healthy Strong People

Good food is one of the four basic pillars of health (along with pure water, moderate exercise, and deep sleep) and the vast majority of our food comes from farms. How the farming business has evolved is inextricably linked to our health. In the years immediately following WWII, a major shift away from time-tested, biologically diverse, traditional farming techniques, to practices best described as large-scale mono-cropping, picked up critical momentum. Mono-cropping is the agricultural practice of growing a single crop year after year on the

> **Exhausted soils cannot grow healthy, nutrient-rich food, so the real work of organic growers is the building and nurturing of strong, healthy soil.**

23

same land. Corn, soybeans, and wheat are commonly grown in this way. Economically, this is very efficient because it allows for specialization of equipment, skills, training, and technologies.

However, mono-cropping has serious negative impacts. It invariably damages the soil ecology by depleting or significantly reducing the diversity of soil nutrients. And because opportunistic insects and weeds are given repeated chances to adapt to the same pesticides and herbicides year after year, mono-cropping increases crop vulnerability. The result is a more fragile ecosystem with an increased dependency on pesticides and artificial fertilizers.

Farming in the late 1940s and 50s also incorporated widespread re-purposing of petrochemicals used in war-time, into pesticides, herbicides, and insecticides, as well as highly resource-intensive techniques like large-scale irrigation. American agriculture has remained firmly entrenched in these relatively untested, artificial, modern techniques ever since. **Chemical fertilizers, pesticides, herbicides, topped off with preservatives and additives for taste and appearance in the end products, have become the *new normal* in our food supply.**

But, do these methods work? That depends on your definition of "work." During the last 60 years, those short-sighted, profit-driven farming methods have "worked" to destroy over 50% of the topsoil needed for food production. We tend to think of soil as a renewable resource - one that is constantly being replenished by decaying matter. But modern farming methods are causing the US to lose topsoil 10 times faster than the natural replenishment rate. Agricultural decisions made for economic reasons alone are proving disastrous. Compare this to the natural farming methods that were employed for thousands of years, leading to the preservation of this precious renewable resource for future generations.

Think of a present day organic farmer, and you'll likely conjure up an image of a guy with an unkempt beard, sandal-clad dirty feet, and a bio-diesel Volvo wagon. That wasn't always the case. Some who appreciated the value of strong soil were jacket-and-tie mainstream types. Back in the 1930s, when modern farming techniques began putting our nation on the brink of a food crisis, top government officials, in fact *the* top government official, **President Franklin Delano Roosevelt demonstrated his surprisingly holistic understanding of large scale agriculture when he famously said, "A nation that destroys its soils destroys itself."**

While FDR's argument might be controversial today, it should have been abundantly obvious to Americans suffering through the Dust Bowl, which occurred several decades after the Potato Famine in Ireland. Few should have needed reminding of the delicate nature of farming. A US Senate report written, remarkably, in 1936 stated, "The alarming fact is that foods - fruits, vegetables and grains - are now being raised on millions of acres of land that no longer contains enough of certain needed minerals. These foods are starving us - no matter how much of them we eat!" Nonetheless, these warnings went unheeded as mainstream agribusiness rolled forward with increasing momentum.

As food rights activist Peter Rossen further explained: "Farming has become petroleum dependent. Some of the more recently developed seeds will only produce their highest yields if given specific amounts of chemical fertilizer, pesticides, and water. So as the new seeds spread, petrochemicals become a necessary ingredient of farming. Because farming methods that depend heavily on chemical fertilizers do not maintain the soil's natural fertility and because pesticides generate resistant pests, farmers need ever more fertilizers and toxic pesticides just to achieve the same results."

The Good News Is, Organic Practices Completely Eliminate Those Hazards

Exhausted soils simply cannot grow healthy, nutrient-rich food. So the real work of organic growers begins with the building and nurturing of strong, healthy soil using organic composts, cover crops, manures and well-planned crop rotation. Along with the genetics and quality of the seeds, the nutrient values of harvested food are linked primarily to the biological activity of the microbes, organic matter, and mineral composition of the soil. Nutrient-rich, healthy, strong soil leads to healthy, strong crops. Healthy, strong crops lead to healthy, strong people.

Probably the biggest misconception about growing organic vegetables is that many people mistakenly believe that the only thing organic farmers and gardeners do is forgo the use of toxic chemical herbicides and pesticides. However, that's only one small part. **Real national healthcare should start with, reestablishing and protecting healthy soil. That is the foundation of sustainable health.**

When synthetic forms of nitrogen, phosphorus and potassium are applied topically, rather than being organically generated through time-tested farming practices, they are easily flushed out by wind and rain. Plus, modern farming methods typically add only a few minerals that help crops grow large quickly, while over 70 elements are needed for optimum human health. In order for these elements to be present in our food, they must first be present in the soil (and/or water). Organic soil-building methods naturally help to fully enhance and restore soil. In short, organic soil has more of the "good stuff" to start with and hangs onto more of it for a longer period of time, while synthetic chemical-based systems lose the "good stuff" more quickly. It's the good stuff (a diverse supply of macro and micro minerals) in our food that helps us enhance and maintain our health.

When considering health and environmental issues, long range thinking is paramount. The Iroquois Indian Tribe's philosophy of seven generation sustainability posits that it's appropriate to think seven generations ahead and decide whether decisions made today would benefit children seven generations into the future. *"In every deliberation, we must consider the impact on the seventh generation ...even if it requires having skin as thick as the bark of a pine."*

Jeff Moyer, Rodale Institute Farm Director wrote: "Even a poor or damaging system can be sustained for a short time. In only seventy years, our current chemical-based agricultural system is already showing major weaknesses - depleted soil, poisoned water, negative impacts on human and environmental health, and dysfunctional rural communities." We should be directing our valuable time and resources to working towards a truly sustainable food production system based on sound biological principles. Numerous studies have begun to capture the true extent of how our low-level exposure to pesticides could be quietly, yet inexorably causing serious health problems in our population. Our disappearing topsoil isn't the only casualty of modern farming.

Toxins from modren farming methods are nearly inescapable. **More than 17,000 pesticide products are currently on the market. Those pesticides are by name, definition, and purpose, designed to kill.** Humans living in farming areas are often exposed to significant amounts of dozens of different pesticides not only in their food but in the air and groundwater as well, it's an inescapable part of conventional modern farming. Exposure to these chemicals has been linked to brain/central nervous system disruption, breast, colon, lung, ovarian, pancreatic, kidney, testicular, stomach, and other cancers. Pesticides (including ones that have been banned for years) have been recently found in breast milk and umbilical cord blood. I believe the human species long-term survival will ultimately depend on us re-learning to exist without exposure to these toxins.

Michael Pollan, author of <u>The Omnivore's Dilemma</u>, points out that the unintended consequences of modern farming methods including, tainted soil and depleted aquifers are reasons to look for new strategies. How can we be expected to look out for the seventh generation when we can't even protect the next generation from conventional farming? **And in that sense what's old is new again. Time-tested organic farming methods are the way forward.**

To repair our food system, we must get back to focusing on the basics - soil health and water quality. How we can improve upon these natural resources so that we return as much as we take, thus ensuring our future? Moyer's answer: "By building and improving soil health, utilizing organic practices to fix nutrients in the soil, encouraging biodiversity, and greatly minimizing synthetic inputs, organic producers are ensuring the sustainability of the system indefinitely. We will not just feed the world's growing population today, or tomorrow, but far into the foreseeable future."

In addition to producing more nutrient rich food, strong soils can also produce resilient plants that are less susceptible to environmental challenges. **Results from the 30-year Farm Systems Trial conducted by the Rodale Institute in rural Pennsylvania demonstrated that in years of drought, organic corn yields were 31% higher than conventional farming yields.** These drought year yields are especially remarkable when compared to genetically engineered supposedly "drought tolerant" varieties which saw increases of only 6% to 13% over conventional (non-drought resistant) varieties. Plants grown from healthy soil are also more resistant to pests.

There is ample evidence that foods grown from rich organic soil are more nutritious. In addition, organic farm and garden practices are safer for all aspects of the environment. All living creatures and ecosystems benefit from sustainable organic growing practices - from the soil microorganisms and earthworms, to our children, grandchildren, and pets. Thinking for now, and for seven generations into the future, it's the farming and gardening practices that will create the greatest long-term yield for our health and planet. Organic farming and gardening is the only ethical, intelligent, and healthy choice.

5

GMOs – Profits Over Health Is Monsanto's Farming Model

Roundup The Usual Suspects

When a company spends billions of dollars developing genetically modified organisms (GMOs), why would they then spend millions to prevent the labeling and advertising of their new products? Obviously, it's because they have something to hide. In November of 2013, bio-tech food giant Monsanto spearheaded opposition to a proposed law that would have mandated the labeling of genetically modified foods in Washington state. Opponents raised over $22 million, while supporters raised only $6 million. The bill was narrowly defeated by Monsanto and friends. Passage would have had no impact on the legality of GMOs, just people's right to know what they're eating. Similar scenarios play out, state by state, all over the US.

GMO science is relatively new. It allows DNA from one species to be injected into another species in a laboratory, creating combinations of plant, animal, bacteria, and viral genes that cannot be created by the forces of nature alone. GMOs are created only through the gene-splicing techniques of bio-technology (also called genetic engineering, or GE). They began infiltrating our food supply in the mid 1990s.

Most people still don't understand the basic differences between hybridization and genetic modification. **Natural hybridization is nothing more than a cross between two closely related species – usually two plants**. Hybrids have happened naturally throughout history via cross-pollination. Wind, water and animals are common facilitators in this process. Even when gardeners or farmers help the process along, hybridization has always occurred between two closely related species. In the animal kingdom, an example of a hybrid is a mule, which is a cross between a male donkey and a female horse. Generally, mules are more patient, sure-footed and more willing workers than either parent.

In contrast, GMOs are created in labs by scientists combining organisms from two totally different biological kingdoms that could never be blended by nature alone. For example, Monsanto has crossed genetic material from a bacterial pesticide, Bt (*Bacillus thuringiensis*), with corn. The goal was to create a pest-resistant plant. This means that any pests attempting to eat the corn plant will die since the pesticide is part of every cell of the plant. The resultant GMO plant, known as *Bt Corn*, is itself registered as a pesticide with the EPA. So, if you feed this corn to your cattle, your chickens, or your children, you'll be feeding them an actual pesticide in every bite. Bt could never naturally become part of the corn seed.

GMOs Have Undergone Virtually No Testing To Prove Safety Claims

Even though GMOs have been created for ingestion as a long-term food source for humans, there have been no long or medium-term safety tests done by the US Food and Drug Administration (FDA), thanks to a 20-year-old policy that says it's up to the bio-tech companies to determine the safety of genetically engineered foods. So while all other developed countries set standards to identify and label GMO plants, a government agency in charge of protecting US citizens essentially lets bio-tech companies, who stand to make billions in profits from GMO foods, create their own GMO policies that include "voluntary safety consultations." Rather than allowing humans to be the long-term guinea pigs in this experiment, the FDA needs to step up and do the science now.

On the one hand, bio-tech giants like Monsanto, Syngenta, Dow Chemical and Bayer, argue that the GMO seeds they create are so unique, they deserve to be patented. On the other hand, the same firms argue that the GMO seeds are "substantially equivalent" to other seeds, so there's no need for labeling, testing, or regulation. Looks like Monsanto wants a monopoly on the seeds themselves *and* both sides of the discussion – having their GMO cake and eating it too!

Right now, Americans are essentially swimming blindfolded in a giant test tube at the center of a massive, Monsanto-led, GMO food experiment. I can think of no other class of food products or additives that have so managed to completely escape government oversight.

Monsanto and the US Environmental Protection Agency were adamant the pesticide in GMO corn, Bt, would only affect insects munching on the crop. They claimed Bt toxin, would be completely destroyed in the human digestive system and would have no possible impact on animals and humans.

Both claims were proven dead wrong. In 2012, doctors at Sherbrooke University Hospital in Quebec, found Bt toxin produced by GMO corn in the blood of 93% of pregnant women tested and in the umbilical blood from 80% of their babies.

Ironically, farmers are now discovering rootworms have become immune to the genetically modified corn. In parts of Illinois, Minnesota, and Nebraska, where rootworm has made a comeback, farmers have now returned to using chemical pesticides along with the Bt Corn. So humans, animals and the environment are now getting a double dose of toxins.

Some GMO crops have been created to withstand massive applications of Monsanto's herbicide Roundup (glyphosate). The thinking is that Roundup will kill the weeds and leave the crops standing tall and healthy. **Monsanto's website claims that Roundup is: "a perfect fit with the vision of sustainable agriculture and environmental protection." Further, it claims that using Roundup creates the benefits of, "maximum profit, efficiency and convenience." Nowhere on their site is there any mention of safety concerns or tests.**

Seeds for crops that can withstand massive doses of Roundup are called "Roundup-ready". While the genetically modified crops are resistant to applications of the weed-killing Roundup, farmers are now increasingly having to deal with Roundup-resistant "superweeds." In many cases they are having to apply more pesticides than ever. It is now estimated that in the period from 1996, when the GMO crops were introduced, to 2011, an additional 404 million pounds of chemical pesticides were applied to US fields, amounting to a 7% increase overall.

One of the biggest problems currently is that weeds are becoming resistant to Roundup. But Bob Kremer, a microbiologist with the US Department of Agriculture's Agricultural Research Service said: "research appears to show that repeated use of the chemical glyphosate, the key ingredient in Roundup herbicide, impacts the root structure of plants. The less visible problems below the soil should be noted and researched more extensively." He also said, "our research shows that these genetically altered crops do not yield more than conventional [traditional] crops, and nutrient deficiencies tied to the root disease problems is likely a limiting factor."

Kremer is among a group of scientists who have been turning up potential problems with glyphosate. Outside researchers have also raised concerns over the years that glyphosate use may be linked to cancer, miscarriages, and other health problems in people and livestock.

It's not surprising that Monsanto had no comment on Kremer's findings but has said in the past that glyphosate binds tightly to most types of soil and is not harmful. The company has said that its research shows glyphosate is safe for humans and the environment. It is disturbing that neither the United States Department of Agriculture nor the Environmental Protection Agency, have shown interest in further exploring this area of research.

In addition, the GMO industry claim that their crops can coexist with non-GMOs and remain segregated, is flat out false. They completely ignore the natural impacts of wind, insects, floods, and animals. Corn pollen can easily drift miles in windy conditions (not even Monsanto has figured out a way to control the wind). Peter Thomison of Ohio State University wrote, "even if only a small percentage of the total pollen shed by a field of corn drifts into a neighboring field, there is considerable potential for contamination through cross pollination." The unintended spread of GMO crops cannot be controlled any more than man can control which way the wind blows. Contamination permanently alters a species' gene pool, undermines the ability of organic and other non-GMO farmers to receive fair pay for their efforts and prevents exports to countries that want nothing to do with GMOs. In 2013, this happened when experimental GMO wheat was discovered in Oregon farmland that was supposed to be GMO free. **When the news broke that GMO seeds had contaminated these crops, Japan and other countries refused to buy wheat grown in Oregon.**

It's obvious that when Monsanto talks about "maximum profit, efficiency and convenience" they are speaking for themselves, not for the long-term benefit of the environment or the farmers that they've hoodwinked into using their GMO Frankenseeds.

It's Not Nice to Try To Fool Mother Nature ... Again

In 1944, Monsanto became one of the first manufacturers of the insecticide DDT. The company reported it to be safe because it was not immediately acutely toxic. It was 30 years before the devastating environmental impacts were discovered and acknowledged. Very low, seemingly harmless concentrations of DDT in streams, lakes, and bays, increased in concentration, an astounding 10 million times further up the food chain – 0.000003 ppm (part per million) concentration in water became 25.0 ppm in carnivorous birds like osprey, eagles, and hawks.

High concentrations of DDT caused the birds to produce eggs with thinner shells that cracked easily during incubation preventing the birds from successfully reproducing, nearly making them extinct. It can literally take decades for the effects of environmental toxins to be accurately identified. Thorough testing is of paramount importance.

Applying the lessons learned from the DDT fiasco to the use of GMOs should tell us that we may not currently be aware of possible negative future outcomes from widespread GMOs.

The Fix Is In

On Saturday May 25th, 2013, people in 430 cities in 52 countries participated in the March Against Monsanto. Estimates placed the total number of marchers at approximately 2-million people. My wife and two of our children each marched in their home city, so *we know* the march took place. Why was there virtually no mainstream media coverage?

Could it be the fix is in? After all, President Obama appointed a former Monsanto VP, Michael Taylor, as FDA Deputy Commissioner of Foods. Taylor was also the FDA Deputy Commissioner for Policy in the 90s. The years in between, he was employed by Monsanto as Vice President of Public Policy. Going back to the 1990s, the revolving door between Monsanto's board of directors and the top levels of our federal government has been well documented. When the top democrat in the government sells us out on this issue, we have a huge problem. There is also little doubt where recent presidential candidates Mitt Romney or John McCain would be on this if they had their finger on the GMO button. Both sides of the political aisle have sold out. And they've obviously taken the New York Times, Washington Post, CNN, ABC, NBC, CBS, MSNBC and Fox News right along with them.

Studies have recently been released indicating that GMO crops and Roundup (glyphosate), present serious dangers. Researchers at the University of Caen in France were the first ever to examine the long-term effects of eating GMOs. Amazingly, no such studies were done in the US by the FDA before GMO corn was approved. I attribute that to the power of Monsanto's lobbying (payoffs) in Washington.

The results of the French experiments are extremely disturbing: in male rats there were liver and kidney damage and tumors. Eighty percent of female rats had mammary tumors. Fifty percent of males and 70% of females suffered premature death. Rats that drank trace amounts of Roundup (at levels legally allowed in the water supply) had a 200% to 300% increase in large tumors. Doctors associated with the study said it's reasonable to assume that GMOs would prove toxic to humans as well.

Further, research now demonstrates that those who regularly eat GMO foods may experience increases in inappropriate immune system over reactions - resulting in increased allergies, asthma and even organ damage. An increasing number of forward-thinking US doctors now recommend that their patients stop eating GMOs to begin their treatment for many chronic inflammatory conditions like asthma, allergies and rheumatoid arthritis.

If the mainstream media gave studies like these any exposure at all, it would likely be devastating to Monsanto and other bio-tech companies currently fighting tooth and nail to prevent mandatory GMO labeling. After all, who would knowingly eat foods that are designed in laboratories to actually be pesticides and have been proven to accumulate in and are likely destructive to human bodies?

Common Sense Around The World On GMOs Bypasses The US

In Norway, Austria, Germany, the UK, Spain, Italy, Greece, Luxembourg, and Portugal have GMO restrictions. France has laws that clearly define what GMO-free means on food labels. Ireland has banned all growing of GMOs and the European Union has considered a continent-wide outright ban of GMOs. Numerous Asian and African countries have banned the growing and/or distribution of GMOs as well. So far, a total of 64 countries have laws requiring some type of GMO labeling according to the Center For Food Safety.

The United States produces 72% of the world's GMO foods even though the long-term genetic effects on humans from consuming the new combinations of proteins and in some cases pesticides, produced in GMOs are unknown.

In 2014 Vermont passed a bill into law that will require the labeling of GMOs - making it the first stand-alone GMO labeling law in the nation. After signing the bill into law Governor Peter Shumlin said, "Vermonters take our food and how it is produced seriously, and we believe we have a right to know what's in the food we buy. More than 60 countries have already restricted or labeled these foods, and now one state - Vermont - will also ensure that we know what's in the food we buy and serve our families." Under the new law, food offered for retail sale that is entirely or partially produced with genetic engineering must be labeled as such by July 2016. This is a bold step in the right direction that other states should follow.

Lawmakers in the state of Vermont should be applauded. Instead, the state is being sued by the Grocery Manufacturer's Association, the Snack Food Association, the International Dairy Foods Association, and the National Association of Manufacturers. GMO labeling is about freedom. It allows consumers to make informed decisions about the foods they eat. Information is power, which is why these trade groups, financially supported by the bio-tech industry don't want want us to have it.

For now, your only escape is to grow your own or buy foods that are "Certified Organic." Yet as we learn, the battle lines are constantly being re-drawn. A "Certified Organic" designation today provides reasonably good assurance that the product is GMO-free. The "Non-GMO Project Verified" seal on the package provides even better assurance – both together, is the best. GMO labeling and restrictions would be a blow to the bottom line of bio-tech giants like Monsanto, but would be a win for mankind, now and for all future generations. For a "Wellness Uprising" to succeed, ultimately we will need to definitively win the battle of GMO labeling.

6

Building And Maintaining Healthy Bones

Slick Ad Campaigns For Dairy Products Build Strong Sales, Not Strong Bones

When you think of bones, you might picture a hard, brittle, skeleton hanging in the corner of your high school science classroom. In fact, bones are actually dynamic living organs, with live cells and flowing body fluids. Without strong, resilient bones we humans would be in sad shape. If you think about it, without bones we'd have no shape at all!

Kidding aside, if you want strong, healthy bones, regular weight-bearing exercise is essential. Finding the truth about a bone-strengthening diet, unfortunately means wading through an endless onslaught of slick ad campaigns touting the alleged benefits of dairy food. Commercials featuring slogans like: "Got milk?" and "It does a body good," and cute milk mustaches on celebrities and star athletes, all but promise youthful health, beauty, and fitness. The truth: **the highest osteoporosis rates**

in the world are in North America and northern Europe where we consume the most dairy products. Meanwhile, 98% of Southeast Asians are lactose intolerant, consume no dairy products and have the lowest hip fracture rates in the world. Calcium consumption in Japan is about half of what the US Recommended Daily Allowance suggests - yet their hip fracture rate is less than half of that of people in the US.

Osteoporosis means "porous bone." Bone is living tissue that is continually being broken down and rebuilt throughout our lives. Osteoporosis occurs when more bone breaks down than is formed. In 2004, the Surgeon General issued a warning that osteoporosis

Milk's Possible Cancer Risk

The modern American way of raising dairy cattle is not only a strain on cows but also produces milk that is unnaturally high in estrogen. Excess estrogen can inappropriately feminize tissues, cause early sexual maturation in young girls and feed certain kinds of cancer.

In the United States, the typical dairy cow is often milked while pregnant. This is made possible because she is impregnated by artificial insemination while still producing milk from her previous birth.

Milk from pregnant cows has higher hormone levels than milk from non-pregnant ones – five times the estrogen during the first two months of pregnancy, and up to 33 times as much estrogen as the cows get closer to term.

(the most common type of bone disease) could reach epidemic proportions by 2020, if action is not taken. The cost of weak bones to Americans, their families, and the country is huge. The medical expense for treating broken bones from osteoporosis is approximately $18 billion each year. The cost of aftercare for these patients and lost work adds billions more.

And what if you're one of those people who breaks a bone? Healing time increases as we age, and if you are elderly, a broken hip makes you to be up to four times more likely to die within three months. One in five people with a hip fracture ends up in a nursing home within a year, according to that Surgeon General report. So the question becomes, what is the correct action?

In a 12-year Harvard study of 78,000 women, those who drank milk three times a day actually broke more bones than women who rarely drank milk. Similarly, a 1994 study in Sydney, Australia, showed that higher dairy product consumption was associated with increased fracture risk: those with the highest dairy consumption had double the risk of hip fracture compared to those with the lowest consumption. Got milk?

The amount of calcium in your bones is one measure of how strong they are. In addition your muscles and nerves *must* also have calcium and phosphorus to function properly. If these minerals are in short supply from foods you eat, your body simply takes them from your bones and teeth.

Each day calcium is deposited and withdrawn from your bones. Our blood pH needs to measure a slightly alkaline 7.4 for body systems to function properly. If our blood becomes too acidic (low pH), calcium will be leached from the bones into the bloodstream (as a survival mechanism), to maintain healthy pH so chemical reactions in our bodies can continue normally. Factors that can contribute to making your blood too acidic include:

- ⅄ Over consumption of sugar or alcohol
- ⅄ Over consumption of animal protein, if insufficient vegetables are eaten as a complement
- ⅄ Lack of sleep
- ⅄ Excessive stress or worry
- ⅄ Lack of fresh air
- ⅄ Exposure to environmental toxins and many medications
- ⅄ Haphazard food combining (example, citrus fruit is best consumed by itself on an empty stomach)

A general rule of thumb I use is that most things that make your eyes bloodshot are acidifying (excluding irritations localized in the eyes themselves).

Another common detriment to bone health is the over-consumption of soft drinks. The average American drinks 150 quarts of strongly-acidifying carbonated soft drinks per year which creates a negative calcium balance and leeches calcium from our bones. Internationally respected naturopathic doctor (ND), Michael Murray stated that "soft drink consumption in children poses a significant risk which can create an osteoporosis time bomb."

So if you're not getting enough calcium, or if you are inadvertently creating an acidic condition with unhealthy choices, you could be withdrawing more than you're depositing. That's why children and teens need to build their bones early so they have a "savings account" of calcium for later. Our bodies build up calcium in our bones efficiently until we are about 30 years old.

That is when our bones reach their maximum weight and density. Healthy habits can help us retain the level of bone mass we have.

To get the most out of our diet, include foods that provide readily absorbed sources of calcium. Among these are dark leafy greens like collards, kale, and broccoli (not spinach); almonds, almond butter, sesame seeds, tahini and other nuts and especially SEA VEGETABLES - the gold standard for mineral-rich alkalizing foods - which can contain 10 times the calcium of milk. Further, these dark green vegetables also provide raw materials for collagen (another important component of bone) production. These foods are also high in magnesium, vitamin K, and other required trace minerals and are best for building healthy bones. Milk contains calcium but provides insufficient complementary nutrients to help your body synthesize bones.

Beyond eating more vegetables, you can cook meat with the bones for greater balance and digestibility. Traditional cultures will use the entire animal and often cook the mineral rich bones, along with the meat, making the meat less acidifying. When making chicken soup, I first boil the whole bird, then carve the meat off the bones, pressure-cook the carcass for 3-4 hours, puree the carcass in a food processor (everything except the thigh bones - too large), and add the pureed carcass back into the stock. This creates a more alkaline, mineral and collagen-rich stock. Near the end of the soup-making process I cut the meat that was removed earlier, into small pieces and add it back in.

If you don't eat all the vegetables you need, consider using a plant-source, whole food calcium supplement.* Consider only formulas that provide readily absorbable calcium accompanied

---

* I recommend food derived bone health formulas from two companies, Garden Of Life and New Chapter.

by complementary amounts of magnesium, boron, silica, strontium and vitamins K & D-3 – the other nutrients your body needs to absorb the calcium and synthesize strong bones. **Too much of the wrong kinds of calcium (calcium carbonate) that your body is unable to use, can build up and be deposited elsewhere in the body, causing bone spurs, kidney stones and possibly even hardening of the arteries.**

But, to be clear: there is no magic bullet for osteoporosis. If you think that prescription drugs like Fosomax are all you need in the fight against osteoporosis you may wish to think again. If lay people or doctors had the time to analyze clinical trial details they'd find that tests showed this class of drugs provided an "absolute risk reduction" for osteoporosis of only about 1.1%. Side effects like jaw bone death (osteonecrosis of the jaw), are shown to be around 4%. **In essence, Fosomax provides a 1% chance of upside gain versus 4% chance of downside risk. I wouldn't put my money on those odds in Las Vegas.**

When scheduling a dental implant for my wife to replace a back tooth, her dentist asked if she had ever used Fosomax. He wanted to know up front what he might be getting into as far as her jaw bone health.

It should be clearly noted that while drugs in that class may help produce increased Bone Mineral Density (BMD) measurements, they do not appear to be particularly relevant to overall bone health or an accurate predictor of fracture resistance. Dense bones are not necessarily more fracture-proof than less dense bones. Bones are made mostly of collagen, a protein that provides a flexible framework, and calcium, a mineral that gives bones hardness and vertical strength. Calcium supports your weight while you're walking or running. But calcium is a lot like chalk. It can support many times its weight while in a vertical position, but snaps easily with pressure from the side or when dropped. **The combination of calcium *and* collagen makes bones strong *and* flexible enough to withstand real-world stresses.**

Half of all hip fractures occur in women who are not osteo-porotic, based on BMD measurements. Nonetheless, fracture prevention efforts have been focused almost exclusively on BMD, and on drugs and/or supplements that increase it. Large numbers of women visit our store after they've been told by their doctor that they have osteopenia. Osteopenia refers to bone den-sity that is lower than normal peak density but not low enough to be classified as osteoporosis. The doctor's implication is invari-ably that something must done to prevent further "problems." However it's quite likely that what the doctor has measured is simply the fact that a 60 or 70 year-old woman has less dense bones than a woman in her 30s or 40s – not that she is truly at risk for fractures.

Peak bone mass is achieved in early adulthood and then begins a very slow decline. Despite the dairy industry's annual 180 mil-lion dollar advertising budget, milk just doesn't cut it. The most effective strategy to prevent bone loss includes some form of weight-bearing exercise like walking, lifting light weights, tai chi, chi gung or yoga, combined with a strong, calcium-rich diet, with plenty of alkalizing, collagen-enhancing vegetables to help you maintain healthy bone mass and flexibility as you get older. Remember: our bones are designed to carry us through a lifetime. With proper nutrition and exercise they will.

7

Saturated Fats Are Very Good For You

Bring Back The Butter

Throughout history, virtually all cultures around the world have thrived using naturally saturated fats as dietary mainstays, especially for cooking. Butter in Europe, ghee (clarified butter) in India, beef tallow in America, palm oil in the tropics and pork lard in China, are all high in saturated fats. The Inuit and Eskimos eat diets that include large quantities of animal fat, but have very low incidence of heart disease. The Maasai people in Kenya are known for eating huge quantities of saturated fat - sometimes a half a pound of butterfat or several pounds of meat a day - yet their hearts are clean as a whistle!

The fact is, heart disease was extremely rare until about 70 years ago. Around that time the rate of heart disease soared after we began switching away from naturally saturated fats and started relying on man-made hydrogenated fats and polyunsaturated fats. In the US, this began during the Great Depression of the 1930s when we switched from butter to margarine and began using Crisco, a man-made saturated fat derived from vegetable oil, because they were cheaper.

Before 1900, heart disease affected about 8 percent of the American population. By 1950, it caused 25 percent of all deaths. The death rate from heart attack and vascular diseases continues to increase and the two causes combined now account for over 30% of all deaths in the US. During this time, consumption of butter, which is high in saturated fats, fell from over 18 lbs. per person per year in 1900, to about 10 lbs. per person per year by 1950. Today, butter consumption is even lower, yet the rate of heart disease continues to increase.

In the same time span, margarine consumption increased from about 2 lbs. per person per year to 8 lbs. per person per year. If saturated fats are the cause of coronary heart disease, one would expect the rate of heart disease in America to have fallen over the past 100 years, rather than to have increased so dramatically. Similar heart disease patterns have taken place throughout the world in more recent decades. Whenever the population reduces its consumption of saturated fats and switches to polyunsaturated vegetable cooking oils, the rate of heart disease climbs.

Unfortunately, the so-called "proof" that saturated fats are bad for health was widely cited in the 1953 "Seven Countries Study" by Dr. Ancel Keys. In this severely flawed study, he showed that countries where people consumed the largest amounts of saturated fats had the highest rates of heart disease. The biggest problem with the "Seven Countries Study" was that it began as a *22 country study.* Keys cherry-picked the data from only 7 countries that supported his own theory and left out the rest. When all the data is examined in its entirety, it shows that in most countries where people ate plenty of naturally occurring saturated fats, they had low rates of heart disease.

Beyond Keys' lazy, misleading, and probably unethical process, he failed to distinguish between naturally occurring saturated fats and man-made saturated fats (aka trans-fats) that are produced by hydrogenating vegetable oils.

Naturally saturated fats are actually ideal for cooking and baking because they are extremely stable so their molecules cannot form chemical reactions where they take on more hydrogen atoms. **They don't form toxic by-products, so natural saturated fats are great for cooking, even under conditions of high heat.**

The layman's explanation of saturated fats is easier to understand - saturated fats are fats that turn solid when they cool down to room temperature, at about 76 degrees. Unfortunately, this idea gives a negative impression that suggests that saturated fats will harden up inside our bodies. But whether it is solid or liquid, the chemical structure of a saturated fat like butter remains unchanged - just as the chemical structure of water remains unchanged whether it is in the form of ice, water, or steam. Plus, live humans naturally run at 98.6 degrees, well above 76, the liquification temperature.

When consuming saturated fats from animal-based foods, you need to remember two words: grass fed. Grass is the natural food for cattle and meat from grass-fed, pasture-raised livestock is lower in total fat and calories than grain-fed. More importantly, meat from grass-fed animals has two to four times more extremely beneficial Omega-3 fatty acids than meat from grain-fed animals. Omega-3s are called "good fats" because they play a vital role in every cell and system in your body. (more below.)

In the history of modern agriculture, feeding grain to cattle may well be the most half-baked, illogical decision ever carried out. By feeding cows, sheep, and other grazing animals grain, we've demonstrated a complete lack of understanding of the way those animals are endowed with the ability to convert grasses into foods that humans can digest. They can do this because they are ruminants, which is to say that, unlike humans, they possess a rumen. A 45, or so, gallon (in the case of cows) fermentation tank in which resident bacteria convert cellulose from grasses into protein and fats. Those of us without a fermentation tank don't have that ability.

Further, feeding grain to animals that run food through their "fermentation tank" is a dangerous and unhealthy practice. The sugars inherent in the grains end up feeding huge toxic overgrowths of E.coli and other toxic bacteria in the rumen during the digestive process.

Because meat from grass-fed animals is lower in total fat than meat from grain-fed animals, it is also lower in calories. For example, a 6-ounce steak from a grass-fed steer can have 100 fewer calories than a 6-ounce steak from a grain-fed steer. If you eat a typical amount of beef (66.5 pounds a year), switching to lean, grass-fed beef will save you 17,733 calories a year—without requiring any willpower or change in your eating habits. 17,733 extra calories is enough to add about five unwanted pounds to your waistline.

Traditionally, all beef was grass-fed beef, but in the United States today what is commercially available is almost all feedlot, grain-fed beef. The reason? It's faster, and, thus, more profitable. **Seventy-five years ago, steers were 4 or 5 years old at slaughter. Today, they are 14 to 16 months old. You can't take a beef calf from a birth weight of 80 pounds to 1,200 pounds in a little more than a year on grass.** It requires enormous quantities of corn, protein supplements, antibiotics and other drugs, including growth hormones to induce such a rapid metamorphosis. These are the ingredients that make conventionally raised, feedlot meat unhealthy. **Just the fact that a natural food like meat now has an *ingredients* list should be very alarming.**

Coconut oil is another saturated fat which has numerous health benefits. Studies from the 1930's and another in 1981 showed that Pacific Islanders who receive 30-60% of their calories from coconut oil demonstrated nearly non-existent rates of cardiovascular disease.

Through it all, the healing properties of coconut oil were apparent for anyone who was willing to see them. Back in the 1930's, a dentist named Dr. Weston Price traveled throughout the South Pacific, examining traditional diets and their effect on dental and overall health. He found that those who consumed diets high in coconut products were healthy and trim, despite the high fat concentration in their diet.

Similarly, in 1981, researchers studied populations of two Polynesian atolls. Coconut was the chief source of caloric energy in both groups. The results, published in the American Journal of Clinical Nutrition, demonstrated that both populations exhibited positive vascular health. There was no evidence that the high saturated fat intake had any harmful effect in these populations.

The naturally occurring saturated fat in coconut oil is extremely beneficial and provides a number of profound health benefits, such as:

⋏ Improving your heart health by increasing HDL (good) cholesterol
⋏ Improving brain health
⋏ Boosting your thyroid
⋏ Increasing metabolism
⋏ Promoting a lean body and weight loss if needed
⋏ Supporting your immune system.

In a recent double-blind, 12-week long study, researchers evaluated the effects of coconut oil and soybean oil on the biochemical profiles and waist circumference of 40 obese women, ages 20-40. Belly fat, known as visceral fat, is the type of fat linked to heart disease, diabetes, and stroke, among many other chronic diseases.

Divided into two groups of 20 participants each, the women received a daily supplement of 30ml (about two tablespoons) of either soybean oil or coconut oil. They also followed a balanced low-calorie diet, and walked for 50 minutes per day. The end result?

The coconut oil group demonstrated:

⋏ Increased levels of HDL (good cholesterol)
⋏ Decreased LDL/HDL ratio
⋏ Reduced waist circumference/abdominal obesity

The soybean oil group demonstrated:

⅄ Increased total cholesterol

⅄ Increased LDL (bad cholesterol)

⅄ Increased LDL/HDL ratio

⅄ Decreased HDL (good cholesterol)

⅄ No reduction in waist circumference/abdominal obesity

In addition, of all the vegetable oils, using coconut oil as your primary cooking oil makes the most sense because it's extremely resistant to heat-induced damage. Extra-virgin olive oil, while great as a salad dressing or for other non-heated uses, when exposed to high heat, smokes easily and develops an acrid taste. Its chemical structure makes it susceptible to heat-induced damage.

More About Omega-3's

Omega-3s are considered essential fatty acids, meaning that they cannot be synthesized by the human body, but can be absorbed from food. Omega-3s are most abundant in seafood and certain nuts and seeds such as flaxseeds, chia seeds, and walnuts and in meats. In meats from pasture-raised animals Omega-3s are more abundant than in meats from feed-lot animals. Sixty percent of the fatty acids in grass are Omega-3s. When cattle are taken off Omega-3 rich grass and shipped to a feedlot to be fattened on Omega-3 poor grain, they begin losing their store of this beneficial fat. Each day that an animal spends in the feedlot, its supply of Omega-3s is diminished.

People who have ample amounts of Omega-3s in their diet are less likely to have high blood pressure, irregular heartbeat, and are 50% less likely to suffer a heart attack. Omega-3s are essential for your brain as well. People with a diet rich in Omega-3s are less likely to suffer from depression, schizophrenia, attention deficit disorder (hyperactivity), or Alzheimer's disease.

Another benefit of Omega-3s is that they may reduce your risk of cancer. In animal studies, these essential fats have slowed the growth of a wide array of cancers and also kept them from spreading. Initial research has shown that Omega-3s can slow or even reverse the extreme weight loss that accompanies advanced cancer and can also hasten recovery from surgery.

According to the American Journal of Clinical Nutrition, the conclusion of an analysis of the history and politics behind the diet-heart hypothesis was, that after 50 years of research, there was *no* evidence that a diet low in saturated fat prolongs life. Naturally saturated fats taste good, are good for you, and are what our ancestors thrived on for centuries before fake-fats became big business.

8

Straight Talk About Cholesterol, Statin Drugs And Heart Disease

Drug Company Misinformation Ensures Profits Not Health

Twenty-five percent of Americans over forty-five years old now use prescription statin drugs such as Lipitor, Crestor, Zocor, and others to reduce their cholesterol. If you believe their manufacturers' statements, side effects from statins are rare. **However, misinformation about cholesterol and cholesterol reducing drugs generated by pharmaceutical companies ensures profits not health.**

Let's Review This In Four Parts:

1) **What is cholesterol and why do you need it?**
2) **Who decided what cholesterol levels are healthy or harmful?**
3) **Are statin drugs necessary?**
4) **Are cholesterol-reducing statin drugs safe?**

1) What Is Cholesterol, and Why Do You Need It?

Many people are surprised to learn that cholesterol is essential to human life. Cholesterol is a natural fat that's necessary for multiple body functions. It's a building block for cell membranes and many essential hormones, vitamin D, and Coenzyme-Q-10, which is very important for heart health. Cholesterol is manufactured in the liver and available in our diet. Typically, if we eat more cholesterol, our liver produces less to maintain balance.

Dr. Ron Rosedale, an internationally respected expert in nutritional and metabolic medicine states: "Cholesterol is a vital component of every cell membrane on Earth. In other words, there is no life on Earth that can live without cholesterol. That will automatically tell you that, in and of itself, cholesterol cannot be evil. In fact, it is one of our best friends. We would not be here without it. Cholesterol is also a precursor to all of the natural hormones. You cannot make estrogen, testosterone, cortisone, and most of the other vital hormones without it. No wonder lowering cholesterol too much increases one's risk of dying."

2) Who Decided What Cholesterol Levels Are Healthy or Harmful?

In 2004, the US government's National Cholesterol Education Program panel advised those at risk for heart disease to attempt to reduce their LDL cholesterol to extremely low levels. Before 2004, a 130-milligram LDL cholesterol level was considered healthy (many naturally oriented physicians feel even that number is arbitrary and unnecessarily low). The panel's updated guidelines, however, recommended levels of less than 100, or even less than 70, for patients at very high risk. These extremely low targets are virtually impossible for living humans to attain without using multiple cholesterol-lowering drugs.

In 2006, a review in the Annals of Internal Medicine found that there was insufficient evidence to support the target numbers outlined by the 2004 Cholesterol Education panel. The reviewers were unable to find research showing evidence that achieving these extremely low LDL levels was important and found that the previous studies attempting to demonstrate proof suffered from major flaws.

So how did these excessively low cholesterol guidelines come about? It was discovered that eight of the nine "experts" that made the 2004 recommendations were on the payroll of pharmaceutical companies that manufacture cholesterol-reducing drugs. **It appears to be just another good old-fashioned case of perjury-for-profit.** *Despite this,* the American Heart Association still recommends lowering your LDL cholesterol levels to less than 100.

3) Are Statin Drugs Necessary?

The Inuit and Eskimos eat diets that include large quantities of fat, but have very low incidence of heart disease. The Maasai people in Kenya are known for eating huge quantities of fat – sometimes a half a pound of butterfat or several pounds of meat a day – yet they are known for exemplary cardiovascular health. It's worthwhile to note that the meats eaten by the Maasai are primarily from pasture-raised grass-fed animals. Those meats are higher in Omega-3 fatty acids than most meat produced in the US that is usually derived from grain-fed cattle.

Dr. Dwight Lundell performed over 5,000 open heart surgeries during his career. In his book, <u>The Cure for Heart Disease</u>, he wrote: "Prescribing medications to lower cholesterol and a diet that severely restricts fat intake is no longer scientifically or morally defensible." Instead, Lundell believes that: "without abnormal inflammation being present in the body, there is no way that cholesterol would accumulate in the blood vessel walls and cause heart disease and strokes. Without inflammation, cholesterol would move freely throughout the body as nature intended. It's inflammation that causes cholesterol to become trapped."

Lundell says the biggest culprit causing chronic, low-level inflammation is diet – specifically, regular consumption of highly processed carbohydrates that include sugar and white flour and the excess consumption of omega-6 vegetable oils that are highly processed in many foods to provide long shelf-life.

It appears Lundell is on the right track. **Independent research demonstrates that elevated blood levels of C-Reactive Protein (CRP), an inflammation marker, are more predictive of cardiac risk than cholesterol levels.** A study of healthy physicians, published in the New England Journal of Medicine, was the first to show that relative risk of first heart attack or stroke was directly related to elevated CRP levels. And the Harvard Women's Health Study, which looked at 12 different markers of inflammation in healthy postmenopausal women, found that after three years CRP was the strongest predictor of cardiovascular risk. Being tested for CRP is simple, inexpensive and can be done along with a cholesterol test.

4) Are Cholesterol-Reducing Statin Drugs Safe?

Drug companies claim these drugs are safe; but a recent study published in the Annals of Internal Medicine tells a different story. In the real world, 17 percent of patients taking these pills reported side effects, including muscle pain, nausea, liver problems and nervous system issues, including peripheral neuropathy. The list and severity of acknowledged side effects keeps growing; increased risk of diabetes has just been added.

Two statins, Cerivastatin and Baycol, were banned because they caused severe muscle break down, kidney damage and even death. It's interesting to note those side effects supposedly didn't show up in drug company pre-launch testing. Also interesting is that in the US this one class of drug creates over 20 billion dollars of revenue for Big Pharma annually.

Despite most of the medical community handing out statin drugs like they're Halloween candy, growing numbers of doctors are quite sure that taking statins is a big mistake. The practice of giving statin drugs to otherwise healthy people, in order to inhibit the natural body function of cholesterol production, is being seriously questioned.

There appears to be a paradigm shift coming in the prevention and treatment of heart disease. Dr. Duane Graveline, author of <u>Lipitor, Thief of Memory</u>, suffered bouts of complete amnesia that ended when he finally discontinued use of statins.

Anyone who has been in my natural food store knows I speak with authority about many health-related subjects. I read a lot of health related material but the ultimate source of my authority is the real-world, personal health stories my customers share with me. I do my best not to jump to hasty conclusions. However, when I'm told dozens, hundreds, or sometimes thousands of very similar stories, that effectively confirm each other, I'm comfortable repeating them so we can all benefit from each others experiences.

Hundreds of our customers have extremely similar stories about their experiences with statin drugs. Here are three that are representative:

⋏ A 74 year old male customer using prescription statins experienced alternating foot pain and numbness that was debilitating. He was unable to work in his shop standing up for more than a few minutes a time. Two weeks after discontinuing his statin medication, his foot problems disappeared.

⋏ A 71 year old female customer's doctor prescribed an artificial statin drug to reduce cholesterol. Her doctor also said her carotid arteries were 73% blocked and she would likely need surgery to restore proper blood flow to her brain. For two years she endured round-the-clock pain in her arms, legs and joints that started within weeks of beginning the prescription

Are Their Safe Alternatives To Artificial Statins?

One of our customers was opposed to taking prescription drugs because of the risk of harmful side-effects. Instead, she took an all-natural supplement I formulated called "Cholesterol Control." Her results? Total cholesterol went from 252 to 198. Her bad cholesterol dropped 25%, her triglycerides went down 15%, and her good cholesterol remained excellent.

Hundreds of others report similar results

statins. Within weeks of discontinuing the prescription statins her pain was gone.

⅄ My 80 year old father's story mirrors that of many of our customers. He was using Crestor and experienced overwhelming fatigue, constant muscle pain, particularly in his shoulders and arms, shortness of breath, and chest pain with moderate exercise, constantly running nose, dry cough, raspy voice, and abdominal distress. He consulted with three doctors, a general practitioner, an allergist and a cardiologist who performed a battery of tests. None provided help. He finally discontinued Crestor and in less than a week the symptoms were gone and he felt better than he had in many years.

All three and several hundred more of our customers now use an all-natural cholesterol reducing formula I created and, by any measure, are doing far better than when they used statins – showing similar cholesterol reductions with virtually no side-effects.

Dr. Joseph Mercola wrote in his newsletter that muscle pain and weakness, and rhabdomyolysis (muscle breakdown and destruction) are actually the most common side effect of statin drugs, which is thought to occur because statins activate the atrogin-1 gene, which plays a key role in muscle atrophy.

Muscle pain and weakness may be an indication that your body tissues are actually breaking down - a condition that can cause kidney damage. Statin drugs have also been linked to:

⅄ An increased risk of polyneuropathy (nerve damage that causes pain in the hands and feet and trouble walking)
⅄ Dizziness

⅄ Cognitive impairment including memory loss.

⅄ A potential increased risk of cancer.

⅄ Decreased function of the immune system.

⅄ Depression

⅄ Liver problems, including a potential increase in liver enzymes (so people taking statins must be regularly monitored for normal liver function).

⅄ Increased rate of death from all causes

In almost all cases where our customers are dissatisfied with statin drugs, they are shown alternative natural products that nearly always reduce cholesterol numbers just as well as the toxic drugs they gave up, usually with no apparent negative side effects.*

If you think that heart disease is being caused by insufficient drugs in your diet, ask your doctor if a lifetime of prescription statins is right for you. If you want to reduce cholesterol numbers with pills but want to avoid the risks of artificial statins, learning when to say "No" to your doctor can be a life saving skill. There are effective natural formulas that appear to be far better tolerated, and ultimately safer, than artificial statins. You can also go further and factor in sugar consumption and inflammation markers when deciding how best to reduce heart disease risk.

---

* Although very rare, it's been my observation that the naturally occurring statins in red yeast rice may, in some people, cause side-effects similar to those caused by prescription statin medications. This statement has not been evaluated by the FDA.

9

Staying Fit Without The Gym

Save Time and Money By Exercising Common Sense Along With Your Body

Americans are drawn to extremes. When it comes to physical activity, we are prone to regularly scheduled bursts of intense work-outs, yet at other times, we'll consciously and even subconsciously try to avoid a single extra step that might cause the slightest heart rate increase.

Visit virtually any health club and you can observe this phenomenon in action. Often the club exercise bikes are full, while people wait in line for their turn on them. Meanwhile, outside, the club's bike rack will likely be completely empty – and the parking lot will be full of cars. With few exceptions, the parking spaces closest to the club's front door are the ones that fill up first. We avoid free exercise on our way to paying for exercise. If you belong to a health club, you know that I'm not making this stuff up.

The extent of the walking done by many golfers today begins when they get out of their cars in the course parking lot, and

ends when they take their seat, two minutes later in a golf cart. Those golfers are so close to honest-to-goodness cardiovascular exercise it almost makes them sweat. For some reason we tend to compartmentalize, instead of combining the activities we engage in. Between work, exercise, kids, and social lives, there are barely enough hours in the day to isolate each and every part of our day *and* still get the sleep that we need to be healthy.

Americans spend $60 billion annually on fitness and weight loss products and programs. Approximately $2.6 billion of that is spent on gym memberships alone, which leads to separating our physical activity from the rest of our lives.

Could There Be A Better Way?

The Journal of the American Medical Association published the results of a study demonstrating that the simple lifestyle change of biking to work was just as effective in increasing cardiovascular health as a structured exercise program, even for previously sedentary adults.

The US Department of Transportation found that a typical adult who used active transportation had fitness levels of someone ten years younger than their actual age. A 30 minute walk or bike ride is associated with better mental health for men and reduced risk of breast cancer for women, reported the Journal of Epidemiology. In California, people who walked or biked for transportation took 15% fewer sick days than people who commuted by car.

The *Scandinavian Journal of Medicine* conducted a one year study that demonstrated significant cardiovascular improvements in people who biked to work as little as three times per week, two miles each way. Total cholesterol and blood pressure decreased and good cholesterol increased. That test group was average healthy adults, but similar results have been achieved with tests involving the obese.

In the United States 50% percent of trips taken by car could be covered on a bike in 20 minutes or less and 25% could be covered by a twenty minute walk. The time it takes to get into your car, wade through traffic, and find a parking spot, is significant, even for short trips. Now examine the time (and money) you spend at the gym exercising (without actually getting anywhere). Eureka! By combining your workout needs with your transportation needs, you'll find that "active transportation" can make you fit *and* save you time and money.

A 2008 study by the *Journal of Physical Activity and Health* revealed that countries with the highest levels of active transportation had the lowest obesity rates. That alone isn't surprising. But what is cause for great concern is that, increasingly, American parents are putting our country's children on a path to obesity. In 1969, 42% of kids walked or biked to school and obesity rates hovered around 5%. Today, those numbers have changed dramatically for the worse, as just 16% percent of American children walk or bike to school and close to one in three American kids are obese. In addition, 35% are at risk for Type 2 diabetes. The reality is that obese children are far more likely to be obese adults. I've been to dozens of youth soccer games where not a single player or parent has arrived on foot or by bike. It's sadly ironic.

This is not exclusively an attempt to inspire couch potatoes to exercise. Primarily, I am trying to convince those who are already physically active to begin exercising common sense along with their bodies.

For you, your children, and grandchildren the time is now to begin incorporating long-term lifestyle changes that are basically free and, with ongoing participation, will yield benefits forever. Study after study shows that walking or biking to work, play, sporting events, or church will drastically improve your health. The Peninsula College of Medicine confirmed that exercising outdoors in the natural environment not only burns calories and builds fitness, it's also linked to greater feelings of revitalization and increased energy, along with decreased tension, anger, and depression *compared with* exercising indoors. So imagine the good that could come from trading what is likely the most stressful, tense – and possibly expletive-filled – part of your day (your car commute), for what could be a healthy, invigorating walk or bike ride?

There are plenty of legitimate obstacles to active transportation. You may live too far away to avoid driving. Or, you may need to use a car to take your kids to school, to after school practice, or to help you transport a week's worth of groceries. That's understandable. I'm not suggesting you sell your car and buy a $4,000 carbon fiber bike for your ten mile commute. Active transportation isn't an all or nothing proposition. It's simply a goal with a flexible finish line. You walk or bike when it's reasonable. Maybe next time you're shopping downtown you can park your car once and walk to and from multiple destinations for errands and shopping, instead of making four or five small car trips. You may find that the exercise, the fresh air, and the friends and acquaintances you'll encounter on your way, are an enriching part of your day.

I'm currently in my 33rd year of year-round bicycle commuting. In 2009, I only put two tanks of gas in my car the whole year and have saved tens of thousands of dollars in the last three decades by relying on pedal power. **Going to work I don't need coffee to wake up or to jump start my heart and brain; the fresh air and exercise does that. The evening ride home helps calm and clear my mind, so it's reasonable to say that my recreational "drug" of choice has two wheels and hand brakes.**

Even if you are currently a couch potato, taking up the money saving activities of walking or riding to work is likely to make you healthier. My wife and I frequently walk to local restaurants when dining out. One thing is sure: by exercising to and from dinner, we can enjoy more dessert, with less guilt. Walking and riding are easy, fun, and practically free – plus there is no membership or spandex required. What more could anyone ask for?

Spring and summer are the seasons when it's really inviting to break out of old habits. Our daily routines can easily be adjusted to include lifestyle changes that will keep us fit and save money. It gets light early and dark late and the summer weather is practically begging us to be exercising outdoors, alone or with your friends and family. It's a perfect opportunity to undertake healthy habits. You might even get hooked and decide to continue exercising common sense along with your body, year- round. And if you don't, certainly fair weather active transportation is far better than no active transportation.

10

Avoiding The Silent Killer

Healthy Alternatives to Prescription Blood Pressure Medications

It is estimated that one in three adults in the US have high blood pressure. Also known as hypertension, it's often called "The Silent Killer" because many people have it for years with no obvious symptoms. The death rate in the last decade due to hypertension has risen about 20%. The only way to know for sure if you have it is to measure for it.

Blood pressure readings are expressed as two numbers, like 120 over 80. The first number, or systolic pressure, is the pressure when the heart contracts. The second number, or diastolic pressure, is the pressure when the heart relaxes. While many believe that 120/80 is ideal, blood pressure naturally rises some with age and a reading of 140/90 for a 70 year old is in the high-normal range and probably no cause for alarm.

Fortunately, you don't need a doctor to measure your blood pressure; you can easily measure it yourself at home. Accurate, easy to use, blood pressure monitors are available for about $40. Since blood pressure naturally fluctuates, taking readings throughout the day is really the only convenient way to get an accurate assessment. Keep a log you can share with a health practitioner if that becomes necessary. In addition, many people have "white coat syndrome." As soon as they see the doctor's white coat, they get nervous and their blood pressure rises. So taking it yourself throughout the day is generally going to provide the most accurate readings.

Most commonly, doctors treat hypertension with prescription drugs that can have a myriad of possible, negative, short- and long-term side effects. There are three basic types (and a few others) of blood pressure medications: diuretics, beta-blockers, and ACE (angiotensin converting enzyme) inhibitors. Each type has its own list of possible side-effects - some being fairly common.

Diuretics flush extra water and sodium (salt) from your body and may cause these side effects:

⅄ Extra urination. Extra water out means more time in the bathroom. Take these medications earlier in the day and when you're not far away from a bathroom.

⅄ Erection problems in some men.

⅄ Weakness, leg cramps, or fatigue. Diuretics may decrease the body's levels of the mineral potassium, which can lead to these side effects. Certain potassium-sparing diuretics do not have this effect, however.

⅄ Intense and sudden foot pain, which is a symptom of gout. This is rare.

Beta-blockers make your heart beat less forcefully and more slowly and may cause these side effects:

⅄ Asthma symptoms
⅄ Cold hands and feet
⅄ Depression
⅄ Erection problems
⅄ Insomnia and sleep problems

ACE Inhibitors block formation of a hormone that causes blood vessels to narrow, so vessels relax. ACE inhibitors may cause the following side effects:

⅄ A dry, hacking cough that doesn't go away
⅄ Skin rash
⅄ A loss of taste

Clinical research confirms what many of our customers have told me: When it comes to treating and preventing hypertension, one-size definitely doesn't fit all. Formerly overweight customers said they've reduced their blood pressure 20-30 points just by losing weight. Some say they've reduced blood pressure significantly by doing 30 minutes cardiovascular exercise three or more times a week. Others rely on natural supplements to stay safe. Some do all three. There are many ways to create natural balance in our body systems.

Beyond prescriptions (and their potential accompanying side-effects), the most impressive blood pressure reductions I've witnessed are from people who have been able to substantially reduce their blood pressure simply by engaging in relaxation-response breathing and mind techniques associated with tai chi, chi gung, or yoga. These ancient therapeutic exercises usually involve body movement but focus as much on the internal aspects of energy movement and balance. They are usually practiced with the target being improved health of the body and mind through balancing the body's energy (Chi).

One of my teachers, tai chi master Dr. B.K. Frantzis stated: "If there was just one thing I [he] could teach Americans to improve their health, it would simply be to teach them how to breathe." I have taught tai chi and chi gung for 20 years **One of my chi gung students reduced her blood pressure 47 points after just two days of practicing stress reducing breathing techniques.** Reductions of 10-20 points are fairly common. Scientific studies confirm that practicing tai chi or chi gung movements along with their associated breathing techniques has proven to be effective in reducing blood pressure. For full benefits, it's important to find an instructor who understands the soft and relaxed (yin) aspects of these arts.

Often overlooked by Western medical practitioners, an important aspect of healthy blood pressure is the flexibility of the blood vessels themselves. Yoga, tai chi and chi gung are very helpful for regaining youthful flexibility. The cardiovascular system is not simply a machine (your heart) pumping blood through inanimate, rigid pipes. The one-way, flexible valves in the leg veins play an important role in reducing strain as your heart tries to pump blood against gravity, up from your feet. These valves prevent backward flow of blood between heartbeats. If backward leakage occurs, the heart has to work harder to increase the pressure enough to force the blood up.

Common medical advice for healthy blood pressure includes the following factors:

⚐ Normalize weight: The greater your body mass, the more pressure there is on the artery walls.

⚐ Exercise: Lack of physical exercise can increase heart rate and blood pressure.

⚐ Relax: meditation, tai chi, chi gung, and yoga, breathing exercises, and biofeedback can help lower blood pressure.

⚐ Eliminate tobacco use: Nicotine raises blood pressure by constricting blood vessels.

⚐ Reduce caffeine intake: Caffeine increases adrenaline, the fight or flight hormone, which constricts blood vessels. Caffeine has been used to induce panic attacks in clinical experiments. Anything that can cause a panic attack is practically guaranteed to raise blood pressure.

⚐ Reduce Alcohol consumption: Shortly after consumption, alcohol can reduce blood pressure slightly. However 12-15 hours later blood pressure is often higher.

⚐ Avoid processed foods: These are the biggest sources of sodium in today's diet.

⚐ Medications: Some prescription drugs, including steroids, birth control pills, decongestants, NSAIDS, and diet pills can raise blood pressure. Some over-the-counter medicines, such as those containing licorice root, ephedra, ginseng or yohimbe, may also raise blood pressure. Guarana, kola nut, and yerba mate are often included in weight loss formulas and are hidden sources of caffeine that can raise blood pressure.

Natural dietary supplements have been proven to help reduce blood pressure. Natural approaches will likely require more time to show results than prescriptions - generally one to three months should be sufficient to know if they are working for you. In contrast, prescriptions may begin to show results in as little as a few hours. I have seen people in my health food store looking for natural blood pressure help who said their blood pressure was 240 over 120 just from walking around. I always suggest people with blood pressure that high go immediately to see a doctor for emergency treatment and come back when their blood pressure is out of the life-threatening range. Extremely high blood pressure like that can cause serious damage to the blood vessels themselves resulting in stroke, heart attack, or kidney failure.

Studies have shown significant decreases in both systolic and diastolic blood pressure among people with hypertension after taking a magnesium supplement for just 12 weeks. **One local customer recently reported reducing his blood pressure 24 points in one week by simply adding a magnesium formula to his fitness regime.** With supplemental magnesium it is important to understand that its complementary partner is calcium, so you should use both. Typically, for blood pressure reduction, you would use at least twice as much magnesium as calcium. That ratio works quite well for most people. The only major negative from too much magnesium is that it can be laxative. Generally it is best to begin with a small dose taken twice per day and gradually build up until you reach bowel tolerance.

The herbs horse chestnut and butchers broom can increase the strength and elasticity of the blood vessels and valves which can help take strain off the heart. **The herb hawthorn** has been shown to dilate coronary arteries, strengthen the heart contractions and reduce blood pressure. **Coenzyme Q-10 (Co-Q-10)** has also been clinically proven to reduce blood pressure. **Customers report that combinations of natural blood pressure reducing supplements often work quite well.**

A team of British researchers recently figured out why **sun exposure** reduces blood pressure. What they found is that nitric oxide stored in the top layers of the skin reacts to sunlight and causes blood vessels to widen as the oxide moves into the bloodstream. That, in turn, lowers blood pressure.

The natural amino acid L-Arginine can increase your body's nitric oxide production. In blood vessels, nitric oxide regulates the tone of the endothelium, the layer of smooth cells that line the inside of the vessels. If these endothelial cells stop functioning optimally, they can cause spasms or constrictions of the blood vessels that can then lead to hypertension. L-Arginine capsules are available in most health food stores.

For some of our customers, reducing or eliminating salt from their diet may have been effective in reducing blood pressure. **However, for many (probably most), a low salt diet seems to have little or no effect.** If reducing salt has virtually no effect on your blood pressure, you are not alone, and there may not be much reason to continue following a low salt diet. Instead, focusing on using high quality sea salt that has a relatively high trace mineral content may create better results.

Dr. David Brownstein, the award winning Medical Director of the Center for Holistic Medicine in West Bloomfield, MI, said that his medical training was clear: a low-salt diet was good and a high-salt diet was bad. "In all hypertensive cases, I was taught to promote a low-salt diet. However, my experience with promoting a low-salt diet to treat hypertension was not successful." Brownstein has written several articles and books stating that low-salt diets are *not* associated with a reduction in blood pressure for the vast majority of the population and also may have adverse effects.

Before committing to a lifetime of toxic blood pressure medications you'd be wise to try one or more of the far healthier natural alternatives for maintaining cardiovascular health.

11

Artificial Sweeteners Are
A Genuine Health Threat

FDA Approves The Toxic And Bans The Safe

Obesity rates among adults in the US have doubled in the last 35 years. Many lifestyle factors have changed in that time. Americans spend more time sitting than ever before. Watching TV, sitting at desk jobs, playing video games, and driving are some of Americans' most popular "activities". Another major change to American habits in the last 35 years is that we are now consuming copious quantities of artificial sweeteners and a relatively new fake-natural sweetener, High Fructose Corn Syrup (HFCS). **It is quite likely that along with less physical activity these *never-before-seen-in-the-history-of-man* sweeteners are contributing to Americans losing the battle of the bulge.**

> It's ironic that in comparison to artificial sweeteners, white sugar should probably be considered a health food.

With focused effort, many people are able to lose weight. The question then becomes: how do we keep the weight off? Regular, moderate exercise and eating sensible portions of healthy foods are obviously the cornerstones of maintaining a healthy weight. Can artificially sweetened "diet" sodas and "diet" foods be considered part of a rational and healthy weight management program? The simple answer is, no. **Remarkably, studies show that Aspartame, the most widely used artificial sweetener of all-time often *contributes to* weight gain and has also been conclusively linked to many very serious adverse health reactions.**

Since the patent on Aspartame expired in 1992, it has been sold under an increasingly long list of enticing monikers. That's by design. Hundreds of millions of dollars spent on marketing campaigns attempt to convince you that you are being offered a fresh, new, zero-calorie sweetener: Equal, NutraSweet, AminoSweet, only name and packaging changes differentiate these identical products. The real truth is – they're all the same old toxic Aspartame.

Just how do Aspartame and other artificial sweeteners cause weight gain? *Scientific American* recently ran an article explaining the science behind this phenomenon. Basically, they wrote that when you eat something naturally sweet, your brain releases dopamine, which supplies you with a jolt of pleasure. Your brain's reward center is activated which encourages you to keep eating. The appetite-regulating hormone leptin is also released, which eventually informs your brain that you are "full" and to stop eating, once a certain amount of calories have been ingested.

In contrast, when you consume something sweet but non-caloric (i.e. an artificial sweetener), your brain's pleasure pathway is still activated by the sweet taste, and you're happy to keep eating. But because your body is still waiting for the calories, no leptin gets released, so there's nothing to deactivate your appetite. As a result, your brain is still sending out signals to continue eating.

Like Aspartame, Sucralose (commonly sold as Splenda), was first synthesized in the mid-20th century, but wasn't sold as a sweetener until 1999. It was first discovered in 1976 when a group of UK scientists were actually trying to create a new pesticide. Its chemical structure resembles pesticides more than it does sugars. Since that time it has gained a 62% share of the artificial sweetener market, primarily because Splenda withstands heat better than Aspartame-based products. Because of that it is commonly used in cooked foods as well as raw.

Though Splenda is a much newer product, it's by no means an improvement. A recent Duke University study determined that Sucralose contributes to obesity, destroys almost 50% of healthy intestinal bacteria and will likely cause more weight gain than eating natural sugar. Something tells me we'll be hearing more bad news about Splenda as more studies emerge regarding this relatively new product.

In his "60 Minutes" TV show report, Mike Wallace stated that the approval of Aspartame was "the most contested in

FDA history." The FDA's own toxicologist, Dr. Adrian Gross told Congress that without a shadow of a doubt, aspartame can cause brain tumors and brain cancer and that it violated the Delaney Amendment, which forbids putting anything in food that is known to cause cancer. But, in what is often the typical FDA protocol, the "Golden Rule" takes precedence - the players with the most gold make the rules. Aspartame's golden manu-facturer, pharmaceutical giant G.D. Searle, came out the winner and the artificial sweetener was approved. How could this have happened?

Enter Donald Rumsfeld, the man who served as Secretary of Defense under presidents Ford and George W. Bush. Rumsfeld was CEO, and then President of G.D. Searle between 1977 and 1985. When Ronald Reagan was sworn in as president on January 21, 1981, Rumsfeld, while still CEO at G.D. Searle, was part of Reagan's transition team. This team hand-picked Dr. Arthur Hull Hayes, Jr., to be the new FDA Commissioner. Dr. Hayes had no previous experience with food additives before being appointed director of the FDA.

After Hayes had been installed, Rumsfeld had G.D. Searle re-apply to the FDA for approval to use Aspartame as a food sweetener. One of Hayes' first official acts as FDA chief was to arrange the approval of Aspartame as an artificial sweetener in dry goods on July 18, 1981 - *mission accomplished!* Hayes left his post at the FDA in November, 1983, amid accusations that he was accepting corporate gifts for political favors. Just before leaving office, he approved the use of aspartame in beverages. Hayes then took a position as a highly-paid senior medical adviser with the chief public relations firm advising both the Monsanto and G.D. Searle companies.

Rumsfeld went on to play an instrumental role in the acquisition of G.D. Searle & Company by Monsanto. Upon completion of the deal, Rumsfeld received a $12 million bonus.

Kickbacks and backroom deals aside, by 1995 there were 92 documented possible negative side effects attributed to Aspartame reported by the Department of Health and Human Services to the FDA. Aspartame has brought more complaints to the FDA than any other additive and is responsible for 75% of such complaints to that agency.

Side effects from Aspartame can occur as acute serious reactions or can occur gradually. When they occur gradually over many years, it can be very difficult to pinpoint the cause. The following is a partial list of documented adverse reactions to Aspartame:

- **Eye** and vision abnormalities up to and including partial or complete blindness
- **Ear** problems – tinnitus – ringing or buzzing sound
- **Neurologic** – seizures, migraines, memory lapses, anxiety, Attention Deficit Hyperactivity Disorder (ADHD) in children
- **Heart** palpitations, shortness of breath, and high blood pressure
- **Endocrine and metabolic** – hair loss, low blood sugar, diabetes, severe PMS

Other – insomnia, excessive thirst, fluid retention, leg swelling, peptic ulcers

Additional Symptoms of Aspartame toxicity can include the most critical symptoms of all:

⅄ Death
⅄ Cancer
⅄ Irreversible brain damage
⅄ Birth defects, including mental retardation
⅄ Aspartame addiction and increased craving for sweets
⅄ Severe depression
⅄ Aggressive behavior
⅄ Suicidal tendencies

In one recent study, the health statistics for nearly 48,000 men and more than 77,000 women over the age of 20 were reviewed. They found that men who consumed more than one diet soda per day had an increased risk of developing multiple myeloma and non-Hodgkin's lymphoma. This 22 year study was the longest human Aspartame study of all time. Yet, for unexplained reasons, this association was not found in women. Leukemia was associated with diet soda intake in both genders.

I'm sure it's quite likely that many people can consume Aspartame and other artificial substances with relative impunity. However, it is a virtual certainty that Aspartame is extremely harmful to many, often without them even knowing the cause. Dr. Joseph Mercola offered the following advice if you suspect you are being negatively affected by Aspartame.

The Most Dangerous Food Additive on the Market: Are You Being Affected?

Unfortunately, Aspartame toxicity is not well known by physicians, despite its frequency. Diagnosis is also hampered by the fact that it mimics several other common health conditions. It's quite possible that you could be having a reaction to artificial sweeteners and not even know it, or be blaming it on another cause. To determine if you're having a reaction to artificial sweeteners, take the following steps:

- Eliminate **all** artificial sweeteners from your diet for two weeks.
- After two weeks of being artificial sweetener-free, reintroduce your artificial sweetener of choice in a significant quantity (about three servings daily).
- Avoid other artificial sweeteners during this period.
- Do this for one to three days and notice how you feel, especially as compared to when you were consuming no artificial sweeteners.
- If you don't notice a difference in how you feel after re-introducing your primary artificial sweetener for a few days, it's a safe bet you're able to tolerate it *acutely*, meaning your body doesn't have an immediate, adverse response. However, this doesn't mean your health won't be damaged in the long run.

⅄ If you've been consuming more than one type of artificial sweetener, you can repeat steps 2 through 4 with the next one on your list.

If you do experience side effects from Aspartame, please report it to the FDA (if you live in the United States) without delay. It's easy to make a report — just go to the FDA Consumer Complaint Coordinator web page, find the phone number for your state, and make a call reporting your reaction.

- Dr. Mercola, June 2013

Nature's New Fake-Natural Sweetener, High Fructose Corn Syrup

High Fructose Corn Syrup (HFCS) has been used as a sweetener in soda since the 1970s, but its use as a sweetener (some call it artificial, some call it natural) has exploded in the past decade. **Folksy television ads featuring farmers standing out in their fields, tending to crops, now try to convince us that HFCS is natural because the main ingredient started out in a corn field. That alone, does not make it truly natural or safe.** The take-out container of Thai food in my fridge is also derived from corn. That alone does not make it edible. The process of turning corn into HFCS is chemical, not culinary.

In reality, the American food system is flooded with cheap HFCS because generous federal subsidies to corn farmers create an artificially low price for corn. Fast food chains add HFCS to their "food" because it is cheaper than sugar. It's in everything: the condiments, the buns, the meat, the drinks. The stuff is so ubiquitous it may even be in their napkins, trays and the little paper hats worn by the employees. The irrefutable fact is, it's the commercially preferred sweetener because it's cheap.

Glucose is the form of energy every cell of your body is designed to run on. Every cell uses it for energy, and it's metabolized in every organ. Fructose, on the other hand, can only be metabolized by your liver. Typical white table sugar (sucrose) is a combination of glucose and fructose. HFCS is also a combination of glucose and fructose, but the bond between the glucose and fructose in the two products is substantially different. As a result, they are metabolized quite differently in the body. The glucose-fructose combination in table sugar is actually metabolized more slowly than the glucose-fructose combination in HFCS and ingestion of sucrose causes your body to produce appropriate amounts of the hormone leptin. Leptin signals the brain (by dialing back appetite) that our caloric needs have been met – so stop eating. Ingestion of HFCS does not appear to create the same level of feedback to the brain.

There is no significant caloric difference between the two sugars and excess sugar (sucrose) and HFCS are both problematic. However, the reason HFCS is even worse and responsible for more weight gain than table sugar, despite having similar caloric content, is due to the differences in how they are metabolized. This manufactured fructose combination leads us to overeating, slows fat burning, and ultimately causes weight gain. On top of all that, HFCS can reduce important chromium levels which can contribute to type 2 diabetes.

Fact is, even though regular cane sugar should be used only in moderation, it is still a *far* healthier option than chemical sweeteners or High Fructose Corn Syrup. It's ironic that in comparison to artificial sweeteners, white sugar should probably be considered a health food.

An excellent option for people who want to avoid sugar and also avoid toxic artificial sweeteners is a sweet-tasting South American herb called stevia. Stevia has been used safely by indigenous people for many centuries and was discovered by scientists and businessmen around 1900. It has virtually no calories or carbohydrates, is safe for diabetics, and doesn't cause tooth decay.

The Story Of Stevia:
The Safe, Natural Sweetener Banned By The FDA Right After Toxic Aspartame Was Approved

The story of stevia being banned and then grudgingly accepted by the FDA becomes even more remarkable considering that these events were happening concurrently with FDA approval of Aspartame.

During the 1960s, food manufacturers in Japan were on the lookout for a natural alternative to sugar. They began using stevia in numerous food products, including candies, ice cream, and soft drinks - products that might otherwise have been sweetened with refined sugar or chemical substitutes. By 1988, refined stevia extract commanded a 41% share of Japan's multimillion-dollar market for high-intensity sweeteners-outselling even the highly popular American-made chemical compound NutraSweet (Aspartame).

By the mid-1980s, stevia was ready to debut in the American marketplace, with the Celestial Seasonings and Thomas J. Lipton Tea companies ready to market herbal tea blends using this sweet tasting herb that is natural, nearly non-caloric and is safe for diabetics. Suddenly, due to an "anonymous trade complaint" from a company that did not want stevia made available to consumers (generally acknowledged later as coming from the makers of Aspartame), the FDA banned import of the herb into the US, and initiated search and seizures (complete with armed federal marshals) in manufacturing facilities and storage warehouses.

Claiming the herb as "a non-safe food additive" despite acknowledging it has "been used throughout history," the FDA refused to respond to petitions filed by the American Herbal Products Association and Lipton Tea Company, denying official Generally Regarded As Safe (GRAS) status, even trying to prohibit the petitions from being filed, a routine procedure that does not require any approval. The FDA refused to read or even acknowledge studies indicating safety and benefits of stevia performed in Japan and Germany.

In 1991 the FDA issued an Import Alert for stevia leaves, stevia extract, and foods containing stevia, calling them "unsafe food additives." This prohibited it from entering the US, and again, was not based on any consumer complaints or actual reports of ill effects. Interestingly, the 1991 Import Alert states that stevia has, "been used throughout history," an acknowledgment that stevia should have qualified as a GRAS product.

Amazingly, the FDA then banned cookbooks that included stevia in recipes and ordered that manufacturers inventory of existing books be destroyed. This had a chilling effect for several relatively small companies who didn't have the deep pockets necessary to challenge the FDA in court. Outrage from the ACLU and the media finally leveled that playing field.

Four years later, in late 1995, the Import Alert was revised, stating that stevia dietary supplements could be imported into the US, provided they are not called "sweeteners" or used as "flavoring agents." It was several more years before consistent stevia supplies could be found to stock in our store. The FDA's nefarious actions effectively removed stevia and information about it from the marketplace for 10-15 years.

The relationship between the FDA's role in approving Aspartame for human use as a sweetener, despite it's proven carcinogenic and toxic qualities, and that same agency's ban of a naturally sweet-tasting herb with a several hundred year safe track-record, is extremely disturbing. Once again leading to the conclusion that, in my father's words, "unfortunately the US has the best government money can buy."

There's a reason that despite soaring obesity rates in America, you'll seldom, if ever, see obese people much older than 65 at their grandchildren's soccer games, out in their yards gardening, or even out shopping. It's not because we're naturally losing weight as we age. It's because significantly overweight people don't live as long, and if they do, they're not mobile enough to enjoy the healthy active lifestyles most of us desire. Obesity greatly reduces the mobility and the overall quality of life of the people it affects. Some are now calling obesity a part of the new American *death-style*.

Please remember that a thirst for artificial sweeteners is directly at odds with your thirst for maintaining a healthy weight or a healthy overall condition. It was true in the sixties, when artificial sweeteners first became popular, it's true now, and it'll be true as long as the FDA and United States Department of Agriculture (USDA) continue to enable the makers of artificial sweeteners to push their toxic products on unsuspecting dieters. No matter what the commercials may imply: high-tech, fake sweeteners are not safe, fresh, new, natural, or healthy. They are dangerous and ultimately will undermine your weight and health goals.

12

Managing Stress

How To Relieve Stress and Prevent Adrenal Burnout

Everyone who is independently wealthy, living in a tropical paradise, surrounded by perfect friends and family, without a care in the world can stop reading now. The rest of us would do well to learn how to manage inevitable daily stress - before it manages us.

Our modern lifestyle, sped up by computers, often asks us to accomplish more in a day than is humanly reasonable. Many people's brains are in hyper-drive from sunrise to sundown, and beyond. The schedule of today's working soccer mom is cram-packed like never before. Data from health insurance companies show that three-quarters of all doctor's visits are the result of stress-related ailments and complaints. In contrast, **I've never heard of anyone being rushed to the hospital by ambulance after suffering from a "relaxation-attack."**

The agreed-upon definition of stress is "any real or imagined threat, and your body's response to it." Stress response, or as it's often referred to, the "fight or flight" response, is wired into our genetic code as a survival mechanism. It's not necessarily a bad thing. In the face of real danger, the stress response can make super men or women out of us.

When confronted with a serious threat, nerve and chemical signals tell the adrenal glands to release the hormones adrenaline and cortisol. Adrenaline increases heart rate and blood pressure, while cortisol releases blood sugar. These chemical responses may have served our ancestors well preparing for a death match with a sabre-toothed tiger, but are simply overpowering and outdated for most of our modern daily needs.

Instead of a death match with a ferocious predator, most of us share common sources of modern stress, such as paying bills and worrying about our jobs, taking care of our kids and parents or managing our marriage and health challenges - hardly requirements for daily doses of body-shocking levels of adrenaline and cortisol. However, the brain responds to stress as it always has: by seeing every threat, be it a figure approaching us in a dark alley or an overdue credit card bill, as a "fight or flight" scenario.

On top of each kidney there is an adrenal gland, about the size of a walnut. The adrenals secrete many different hormones that regulate blood pressure, how our body uses food, and the blood-levels of minerals. One of their biggest responsibilities is to provide hormones that create changes (sometimes very rapidly) in physiology when responding to stressful or life-threatening situations. It's ironic that although your adrenal glands are there, in large part, to help you cope with stress, too much stress is actually what causes their function to break down.

The result is that your adrenal glands, faced with chronic low-level stress, become overworked and fatigued from pumping out extra hormones for much longer than was ever intended, from a biological survival standpoint. In addition, the rest of our body simply doesn't know how to respond to this persistent influx of adrenaline and cortisol. The adrenals have not adapted well to modern lifestyles.

Some common factors that put excess stress on your adrenals are:

- ⅄ Habitual reliance on coffee or other caffeine sources for enough energy and stimulation to make it through the day
- ⅄ Chronic overwork, including physical or mental strain
- ⅄ Sleep deprivation
- ⅄ Light-cycle disruption (such as working the night shift or often going to sleep late)
- ⅄ Surgery, trauma, or injury
- ⅄ Chronic inflammation, infection, illness, or pain
- ⅄ Constant exposure to temperature extremes
- ⅄ Toxin exposures
- ⅄ Nutritional deficiencies and/or severe allergies
- ⅄ Consistently engaging in excessive exercise
- ⅄ Harboring feelings of anger, fear, anxiety, guilt, depression, and other negative emotions

Due to the nearly ubiquitous presence of coffee in our society, it's worth focusing further on the effects of its consumption on stress. Americans consume 400 million cups of coffee per day totaling 146 billion cups of coffee per year. Thirty-one percent of people make coffee the most important part of their morning routine, brewing a cup before any other morning behavior. Sixty-five percent of coffee consumption takes place during breakfast hours.

However, caffeine does *not* provide energy - only chemical stimulation. The perceived energy comes from the body's struggle to adapt to stress hormones produced by consuming caffeine. **Coffee is the socially-sanctioned drug of choice and it is useful. It allows millions of people to respond enthusiastically to lives and jobs that they would otherwise have trouble waking up for.**

However, constantly responding to chronic stress has been shown to create many major negative effects on our health, which can include elevated blood pressure, sleep and digestive disorders, reduced immune function, muscle tension and pain, or anger and emotional imbalances. There are literally dozens, and possibly hundreds of ways stress can negatively impact health and coffee can exacerbate almost all of them.

Further, habitual coffee consumption can contribute to long-term over-taxing of the adrenal glands and contribute to burnout. It has been my observation that when people discontinue use of coffee by going *cold-turkey* they usually suffer from headaches for about 3-7 days during the withdrawal phase as the blood vessels in their brains normalize. They may also experience some low-back pain as their kidneys adjust. **Then after a week or two of being substance-free, they almost always experience greater feelings of energy and vitality.** Most habitual coffee drinkers don't go off the substance often enough to know what it's like to live their lives "de-caffed'.

Some stress is a normal part of life and may even be considered constructive – like the excitement of starting a new job, planning for a trip or birthday party or welcoming a new baby into your family. But it still can contribute to adrenal fatigue if taken to extremes – emotional balance is the key.

Often people choose the quick and easy fixes – smoking cigarettes or pot, drinking alcohol, or zoning out for hours in front of the TV – to temporarily numb their nerves, attempting to reduce the effects of stress. But inevitably, poor quality coping methods make the effects of stress worse in the long run. These easy fixes feel good (anesthetized) and provide some short-term "comfort," but they do little to actually dissolve the root of the stress that makes us feel bad and seek comfort in the first place. Also, chronic stress often causes insomnia but the use of prescription sleep aids can actually cause memory loss and prevent us from reaching the deepest most rejuvenating phases of sleep, thereby contributing to more stress the next day.

How chronic stress and adrenal fatigue may manifest in your body

- ↟ You feel tired for no reason, even after a couple of good night's sleep.
- ↟ You have trouble getting up in the morning, even when you go to bed at a reasonable hour.
- ↟ You generally feel rundown or overwhelmed
- ↟ You are constantly irritable and short-tempered with those closest to you
- ↟ You have difficulty bouncing back from stress or illness.

⅄ You crave salty and sweet snacks.

⅄ You feel more awake, alert, and energetic after 6 p.m. than you do all day.

⅄ Reduced libido

Instead of a quick, lower quality fix that only temporarily addresses a few symptoms, here are some suggestions for managing stress in healthy, constructive ways. First we need to remember this is an issue that needs attention each and every day. **It's a lot easier and more cost effective to smooth unwanted "stress footprints" out of wet concrete on a daily basis than it is to remove them with a jackhammer once per week after they are "set in stone." Any of the following activities practiced daily should help keep you managing stress constructively. Daily ... not weekly or monthly maintenance is the key.**

⅄ Go for a daily walk or regularly partake in other exercise that you enjoy.

⅄ Spend time in nature or work in your garden.

⅄ Practice yoga, tai chi, or chi gung.

⅄ Meditate.

⅄ Play with a pet.

⅄ Write in your journal.

⅄ Listen to music.

⅄ Get a massage.

⅄ Soak in a bath or hot tub.

All of these activities can create the desired relaxation response in our bodies without the backlash associated with medications, alcohol or cigarettes. Practiced daily, many of these high-quality choices will also have a cumulatively beneficial effect that will act as an insurance policy against future stress.

High quality relaxation techniques can take some practice. Remembering to do them is the first hurdle. As you become more aware of muscle tension, breathing patterns, and other physical sensations of stress, it will become easier to recognize and these sensations will remind you to address it on an ongoing basis.

A student in one of my Chinese exercise (chi gung) classes amazingly lowered her blood pressure 47 points in two days using a centuries old, stress-reducing breathing technique. Think about the possible long-term side effects and financial costs of prescription blood pressure medications contrasted with the long-term cumulative health benefits of natural, daily, habit and lifestyle adjustments. The choice is a "no-brainer."

From the perspective of Chinese medicine, there is usually a yin and yang component to most high-quality remedies. Correspondingly, from that perspective, treating chronic stress or adrenal fatigue has two components. Stress reduction and management is the yin component. Relaxing (yin) herbs often include: **valerian, chamomile, passionflower, hops, skullcap, lemon balm, lavender, and california poppy.** Long-term, gradual strengthening and rebuilding (tonifying) adrenal function is the yang component. Tonifying herbs, also known as adaptogens, used in balanced, high-quality formulas for strengthening adrenal function often include: **rhodiola, ashwagandha, cordyceps, eleuthero (siberian ginseng), holy basil, and schizandra.**

Many of the best formulas contain herbs from both sides of the spectrum. The beauty of exercises like tai chi, chi gung, and yoga is that relaxing and strengthening are accomplished simultaneously.

In contrast, most Western doctors have little understanding of the balance inherent in high-quality healing. They usually only address half of this issue by treating stress exclusively with prescription sedatives (considered very yin) that have a long list of potential negative side-effects. Long-term use of drugs like Valium, Librium or barbiturates often further deplete energy and motivation and can reduce libido and mental acuity.

Choosing nutrient-dense foods during stressful times can replenish vital nutrients like vitamins B and C that are easily depleted by stress. For energy it's much smarter to snack on bananas, nuts, or a salad with avocado than a bag of Doritos or a candy bar. You'll do your body a big favor re-hydrating with coconut water, fresh vegetable juice, or just pure water rather than a caffeinated soft drink which will increase adrenaline and set you up for a stress and sugar induced crash landing an hour or two later.

In severe cases of adrenal fatigue, reestablishing balance and regaining normal adrenal function can take several months or more. In addition to the the healthy daily stress reducing practices mentioned above, during that time it is very important to control your blood sugar levels. Try to observe the following:

⅄ Eat a small meal or snack every three to four hours
⅄ Eat within the first hour upon awakening
⅄ Eat a small snack near bedtime that includes some protein

⅄ Eat before becoming hungry. If hungry, you have already allowed yourself to run out of fuel (low blood sugar), which places additional stress on your adrenal glands

In between stress-free tropical vacations you can treat yourself well by managing stress every day, in balanced high-quality ways, for a tiny fraction of the cost of a trip to paradise.

13

Sleep Should Be Simple, Safe And Sound

Keep Big Pharma Out Of The Bedroom And It Will Be

Sleep Should Be Simple

For thousands of years, humans naturally allowed the sun and the seasons to determine their sleep-wake cycle. Man is not naturally a nocturnal animal. Nocturnal creatures generally have more highly developed senses of hearing and smell and specially adapted eyesight that allow them to successfully compete for survival in very low-light situations. Without these ultra-keen adaptations, animals vying for survival in the jungle or the woods at night would likely get eaten or starve.

To avoid the dangers that darkness in the wild brings, humans are programmed to be safely tucked away within a few hours of nightfall. Each day, when the sun sets and the temperature drops, our body's pineal gland begins to secrete melatonin,

103

the sleep hormone. Within a few hours, sleep should naturally follow. This natural health promoting cycle (our circadian rhythm) is disrupted by artificial lights, late night TV watching, and computer use. Negative effects from sleep disruptions affect all body systems. Sleep is very important; we spend nearly one third of our life doing it. But even though sleep is crucial to our health and well-being, research shows that relying on prescription drugs to induce sleep is very likely to be counterproductive and dangerous.

A number of critical body functions occur during sleep. Regardless of age (although to a much greater degree in children and adolescents), our pituitary glands pump out human growth hormone (HGH) during deep sleep, stimulating the growth and repair of bones, muscles and virtually all body tissues.

Dr. Charles Czeisler, head of the Division of Sleep Medicine at Harvard Medical School said, "sleep is the third pillar of health, along with exercise and eating well." Sleeping for seven to eight hours a night has been proven to positively impact blood pressure, memory, immunity, mental health, obesity, longevity, and much more, compared with sleeping less than six hours a night.

During sleep, the flow of cerebrospinal fluid surrounding the brain increases dramatically, washing away waste proteins that accumulate during waking hours. Build up of these wastes has been linked to Alzheimer's. This phenomenon has been conclusively observed in laboratory animals by Dr. Maiken Nedergaard, a professor of neurosurgery at the University of Rochester and author of a 2013 sleep study published in the journal *Science*.

Penelope Lewis, director of the Sleep and Memory Lab at the University of Manchester in England, says that during the day our brains observe, see, hear, and learn lots of information. During deep sleep is when we organize it - reinforcing and filing the important and deleting the irrelevant. Many college students know that pulling an all-nighter to cram for a test is not nearly as effective as studying for a few hours a night, then sleeping well and letting the information sink in during the days leading up to the exam – even if the total study time is the same.

As vitally important as sleep is, sleep induced by artificial chemicals is probably not worth the risks. Specialists warn to exercise caution before taking sleep medications. "We're not certain, but it looks like sleeping pills could be as risky as smoking cigarettes," said Dr. Daniel F. Kripke, professor emeritus at the University of California, San Diego, and founder of one of the country's first sleep clinics.

In a recent sleep study, a team of researchers led by Dr. Kripke studied over 33,000 people for an average of over 2.5 years. The death rate for people not using sleeping pills was 1.2% versus 6.1% for people with sleeping pill prescriptions. Even those who used 18 or fewer sleeping pills a year had a 3.6-fold higher death risk than people using no sleeping pills. Kripke and colleagues estimate that sleeping pills are linked to between 320,000 and 507,000 US deaths each year. Often people using sleeping pills have underlying health problems that contribute to their insomnia. However, the increase in mortality rates Kripke observed was calculated after controlling the study to take into account age, gender, lifestyle factors, and underlying health problems.

Kripke also said, **"there's no objective evidence that sleep medications help people perform better the next day. The**

majority of studies show they impair performance the following day."

The FDA recently acknowledged that sleep-inducing sedative drugs containing zolpidem (brand names Ambien, Edluar, Zolpimist, and Intermezzo) created a serious risk of injury due to morning drowsiness. The problem is that no sleeping pill remains in the blood all night, impairing consciousness, and then suddenly wears off the moment the alarm clock goes off. Also, a large percentage of people who take sleeping pills do often get up at night, at a time when the sleeping pill could cause falls or confusion.

Most prescription sleeping pills, when taken at bedtime, will remain in the blood with at least half strength when morning comes. According to Dr. Kripke, almost all sleeping pills produce immediate impairments of memory and performance and there is extensive evidence that sleeping pills, on average, impair performance and memory into the following day. Studies have shown Lunesta is especially likely to produce a few hours of morning impairment, particularly among people over age 60. These side effects are more likely to occur in women, who are generally smaller and metabolize these drugs more slowly than men.

Further, sleeping pills cause people to have more depression. The sleeping pill arm of Big Pharma would like you to believe that insomnia leads to depression, which may be true some of the time. However, the implication that prescription sleep medications prevent depression is simply not true. Controlled trials of four different common sleep medications show a higher rate of developing depression among those given the sleeping pills as compared to those given a placebo.

In addition, sleeping pills can have some very strange effects - often comical, occasionally dangerous. Sleeping pills turn off our brain cells, but not always all parts of the brain to the same degree. There are documented stories of people sleep walking, to their kitchens, preparing and consuming elaborate meals, and waking up with no memory of their nighttime escapades. There have also been reports of people under the influence of Ambien who, while sleeping, walked to their cars, got in, went for a drive and got into serious collisions.

Natural Factors You Can Optimize To Improve Sleep

Sleep in complete darkness - or as close to it as possible. If that's not feasible, wear an eye mask to block out stray light. Little bits of light pass directly through your optic nerve and can signal your brain that it's time to wake up. If you get up use the bathroom in the middle of the night, if possible, avoid turning the light on. A dim red nightlight can help. Red has the least power to suppress melatonin and shift circadian rhythms.

Optimal bedroom temperatures - for sleeping are from 60 to 68 degrees.

Keep regular hours - maintaining a regular bed time and wake time (even on weekends) will reinforce your circadian rhythm.

Avoid caffeine - often an afternoon (or even morning) cup of coffee or tea will keep some people from sleeping well at night. Coffee, as well as less obvious caffeine sources such as soft drinks, chocolate, coffee-flavored ice cream, and tea, must all be eliminated if you have trouble sleeping. Even small amounts of caffeine found in decaffeinated coffee or chocolate may be enough to cause insomnia in some people.

Avoid alcohol - alcohol will make you drowsy; the effect is short lived and you will often wake up several hours later, unable to fall back asleep. Alcohol can also keep you from entering the deeper stages of sleep, where your body does most of its regeneration.

Exercising for at least 30 minutes per day - can improve your sleep. However, don't exercise too close to bedtime or it may keep you awake.

Stress reduction and balancing negative emotions often significantly improve sleep - scientists often find increased blood levels of cortisol, a stress hormone, in people with chronic insomnia, suggesting that these individuals suffer from sustained, round-the-clock activation of the body's fight or flight stress response. This constant state of hyper-arousal can dramatically interfere with normal sleep.

Exercise, laughter, listening to your favorite music, relaxation response breathing techniques, and practicing yoga or tai chi can all dramatically reduce stress levels.

Using a cell phone immediately before going to bed (especially for a long call) - can cause insomnia and may also cut your amount of deep sleep, interfering with your body's ability to refresh, rebuild, and repair itself.

Avoid nighttime drops in blood sugar (nocturnal hypoglycemia) - if you fall asleep but cannot stay asleep more than a few hours, it may be due to your blood sugar falling in the middle of the night. Your brain needs sugar to dream and carry out other functions through the night. When there is a drop in blood sugar, it triggers the release of hormones, including cortisol and adrenalin. They help signal the brain that it's time to eat. While I generally don't advise eating before bed, for some people, eating a small snack that includes complex carbohydrates and protein (like a slice of whole-grain bread with some almond or peanut butter) can help to stabilize blood sugar and facilitate a good night's sleep.

Natural Supplements To Improve Sleep

There are many safe, effective natural supplements that can be very helpful to fall asleep and stay asleep. Formulas containing (separately or together) **valerian, chamomile, passion flower, skullcap, melatonin, GABA,** and others have received hundreds of *thumbs-up* from my customers. GABA can be especially effective in relieving anxiety related sleep problems. **Magnesium-calcium** combinations (with more magnesium than calcium) are also helpful. **Lavender oil** applied to your pillow is often all that is needed for a good night's sleep.

You need quality deep sleep just as much as you need clean food, water and air. If you have trouble getting to sleep or staying asleep, more than once or twice a month, you should engage one or more of the natural sleep aids or techniques offered in this chapter. They are infinitely safer and ultimately far more beneficial than prescription knock-out drugs.

Caution: If you have taken a prescription sleeping pill regularly, eliminating the drug suddenly may induce dangerous withdrawal symptoms such as: anxiety, irritability, panic, insomnia, nausea, headache, impaired concentration, memory loss, depression, seizures, hallucinations, and paranoia.

14

Further Study Of Prescription Antidepressants Is Needed Now

Safe, Effective, Natural Alternatives Are Available

One in ten Americans now take prescription anti-depressants. Antidepressant use in this country by people age 12 and older increased 400% between 1988 and 2008, according to the National Center for Health Statistics. Yet there's little evidence that anti-depressants like Prozac, Paxil, Zoloft, and others, provide any benefit treating mild to moderate depression. "They work no better than placebos," concluded a 2010 Journal of the American Medical Association study, yet unwanted side-effects from anti-depressants can be significant and discontinuing their use is often extremely difficult. Using anti-depressants should not be taken lightly.

To be as logical and clear as possible, let's study this important subject in four basic parts:

1) Incomplete Science Can Be Hazardous To Our Health
2) The Tragedy Of School Shootings
3) Healthy Alternatives To Prescription Anti-depressants
4) A Note On Seasonal Affective Disorder

1) Incomplete Science Can Be Hazardous To Our Health

Marie Curie, the brilliant Polish scientist, became an icon for her discovery of radiation. To this day she is the only person to win Nobel Prizes in two different sciences, chemistry and physics. The impact of her work is so far-reaching we're still just scratching the surface of her pioneering research from the early 1900s. Sadly, Curie died from cancer caused by the radioactive materials she discovered. She saw nothing dangerous about them and carried test tubes full of radioactive materials in her pocket and stored them in her desk drawer, often naively marveling at how they glowed in the dark.

As exceptional as Curie was, you could say she was the victim of her own intelligence - an example of modern science's love affair with "the latest discovery" without much thought of how new materials, technologies, and ideas will interact with life in the physical world.

Another instance where initial scientific study was dangerously incomplete was with a drug patented in 1954. Thalidomide was to be used as a sleeping pill but was soon discovered to help pregnant women with morning sickness. Though never approved for sale in the US, millions of Thalidomide pills were given free to doctors for testing, who then distributed them to pregnant women. It was later discovered that Thalidomide caused heartbreaking birth defects.

In 1988 a new, patented drug was introduced with much fanfare: the antidepressant Prozac. It's in a class of drugs called selective serotonin re-uptake inhibitors (SSRIs). Other drugs in that classification are: Paxil, Celexa, Zoloft, Luvox, Effexor and others. Today, they're often prescribed by general practitioners based only on information provided by drug company representatives. According to Dr. Alice Domar of the Harvard Medical School, all you have to do to be prescribed an SSRI is to walk into a doctor's office and say you are lethargic or not feeling well.

Dr. Lissa Rankin rejects that idea. She told *Psychology Today* that anti-depressants aren't the answer: "As an MD, I've watched too many of my colleagues yank out antidepressant samples every time a patient starts to cry. So on behalf of physicians everywhere, let me apologize for our trigger-happy prescription-writing behavior. I don't mean to diminish the pain someone who is depressed might experience. But tears are healthy. Sadness doesn't always need treatment. And it's important to remember that the pain muscle and the joy muscle are the same. If you can't feel one, you won't feel the other," said Rankin.

Dr. David Healy is founder of an independent website for researching and reporting on prescription drugs. He is a world-renowned expert on anti-depressants, has prescribed SSRI drugs to patients and still prescribes them selectively. He thinks general practitioners are prescribing them in good faith. But according to him: "We are not just using them with people who need to be treated. We've gone way beyond that and are actually making people ill."

2) The Tragedy Of School Shootings

Dr. Healy questions what kind of society we have become, "when increasingly it seems pharmaceutical companies can get drugs on the market which have not been shown to work or which have been claimed to be safe and effective when they aren't."

According to Healy: "Some 90% of school shootings over more than a decade have been linked to this widely prescribed type of antidepressant." Harvard psychologist Dr. Joseph Glenmullen discussing SSRIs said: "We don't know what these drugs are doing to real life human beings. When you look at all the documents, you see a pattern of (drug companies) misleading doctors who then unwittingly mislead patients. This is a betrayal of the public trust in physicians behind the scenes by the drug industry and it must stop."

Senator Henry Waxman concluded it is all about money, not science. "The pharmaceutical industry has systematically misled physicians and patients."

Discontinuance of SSRIs is also a *huge* problem; withdrawal symptoms can be horrendous. Many patients while trying to stop their medications, experience sensations of electric shock or jolts that create intense pain, along with fatigue so intense they can hardly walk or talk. Other withdrawal symptoms include fainting, dizzy spells, insomnia, chest pains, stomach spasms, headaches, racing thoughts, crying spells, nervousness, anxiety, anger and violence. **One young man going through it described it as the sensation of all the panic attacks he didn't have while on the drugs, being bottled up inside of him, and now coming out at an uncontrollable rate.**

The use of SSRIs has been connected to many of the school shootings that have taken place since the 1990s. In Springfield, Oregon, 15 year old Kip Kinkel was withdrawing from Prozac when he went to school and shot 22 classmates, killing two, after murdering his mother and step father in their home. The following website indexes over 50 school shootings, among 4,800 total violent events linked to SSRIs: http://www.ssristories.org/. It is the most detailed source I've found on the subject. It states that irrational school shooting incidents started noticeably increasing in 1988, coincidentally, the year Prozac was introduced.

An honest, unbiased, thorough study on the real impact of SSRIs is desperately needed. These are highly volatile drugs, and it's never too late to right our scientific wrongs.

3) Healthy Alternatives To Prescription Anti-depressants
Natural Supplements, Diet, Exercise, And Exposure To Sunlight Can Significantly Improve Mood

World renowned Medical Doctor and Naturopathic Physcian, Dr. Andrew Weil, expresses serious concern about treatment of depression: "Clinical depression can be triggered by a recent loss or other sad event, but then grows out of proportion to the situation and persists longer than appropriate, affecting your emotional health. While there are many theories about mood disorders, the actual causes of depression remain unclear. The current branch of medicine that addresses depression, psychiatry, is deeply founded in materialistic thinking, and believes that all mental problems stem from imbalances in brain chemistry.

Hence, its total commitment to the use of drugs. While it seems likely that some cases of depression may result from deficiencies or excess neurotransmitters, such as serotonin, it makes equal sense to suggest that mood disorders actually cause disordered brain biochemistry." In other words: which came first, the chicken or the egg?

What are some alternatives for treating mild to moderate depression? Weil suggests the following far safer and effective holistic methods:

Check your meds - "Make sure you are not taking any over-the-counter or prescription medications that contribute to depression. Avoid all antihistamines, tranquilizers, sleeping pills and narcotics if you have any tendency toward depression. You should also be cautious about the use of recreational drugs." The rebound effects from alcohol and marijuana can be especially dangerous for people leaning towards depression.

Never skip a meal - "Keeping blood sugar stable reduces mood swings." Smaller, more frequent meals with a little higher protein and fat help stabilize blood sugar.

Cut caffeine - "Addiction to coffee and other forms of caffeine often interferes with normal moods and brain serotonin levels."

Reduce your intake of sweets - "Sweets temporarily make you feel good as blood sugar levels soar, but may worsen mood later on when they plummet."

Eat a serotonin-enhancing diet - "Wild salmon, sardines, herring, mackerel, and anchovies, which are even higher in Omega-3 fatty acids than other fish."

Acupuncture - "Proven itself to be very useful in treating several mood disorders, including depression."

Further, Dr. James S. Gordon, world-renowned expert in using mind-body medicine to heal depression, said: **"Research shows that physical exercise is at least as good as anti-depressants for helping people with mild to moderate depression.** Physical exercise changes the level of serotonin in your brain." Thirty minutes of mild to moderate cardiovascular exercise three or more times per week, should do the trick.

These natural supplements are shown to help elevate or stabilize mood:

B-vitamins - especially B-6 and the L-methylfolate form of folic acid, recommended by southern Oregon physician, Dr. Robin Miller, are proving to be effective for mood-enhancing.

St. John's Wort - is an herbal remedy that's long been used in Europe for treating mood disorders. St. John's Wort is not a quick fix. Full effects are generally felt in 6-8 weeks. Standardized extracts have shown to surpass Prozac for treatment of mild to moderate depression. St. John's Wort has also been shown to be an immune system enhancer with significant anti-viral properties.

SAM-e - pronounced "sammy," is one I'm especially impressed with. It's a natural chemical that is found in the human body and is believed to increase serotonin and dopamine. It can boost mood and help people feel more alert and motivated. I've observed that results are often experienced in as little as a few hours to a few days, making it ideal to use on an as-needed, short-term basis. Although full results may require 4 weeks use. Dr. Weil recommends 400-1,600 mg a day on an empty stomach.

Theanine Serene with Gaba, and Relora from Source Naturals - is a formula that is proving to be a powerful synergistic, natural blend that helps to greatly reduce anxiety and to calm and stabilize moods. It helps provide a sense of mental and physical relaxation.

Dr. Rankin also sees depression in some cases as somewhat self-induced. **She suggests that we make efforts to bolster our mental health by: "being more authentic in all aspects of your life.** Too often, people walk around wearing masks, pretending to be something we're not. We fake it at the schoolyard, in the boardroom, in the bedroom, and at church - and then we wonder why we wind up depressed. Practice letting your "freak flag" fly and watch how your mood lifts."

Sometimes going on a two-week "news media fast" should be just what the doctor orders. Obsessing or dwelling on negative news coverage of deceit, killings, or disasters, can be very disheartening. **Focusing on unfortunate situations *you have no*** *control over* **can create an extra dose of anxiety that no one needs - why go there?** Instead use that same time every day for walking, gardening, listening to music, playing with a pet, or whatever you enjoy doing. A "news fast" and avoiding discussions with people who obsess over negative news are probably the simplest actions you can take to boost mood and improve your outlook.

4) A Note On Seasonal Affective Disorder

Seasonal Affective Disorder (SAD) is usually defined as a type of depression that occurs at the same time every year, usually winter. People living in darker Northern latitudes typically suffer from SAD at ten times the rate of those in sunnier, more Southern latitudes. It's interesting to note that among the Northern countries, those with the highest per-capita fish consumption have the lowest rates of SAD. Eating cold water fish enhances serotonin and cold water fish contain large amounts of vitamin D, the sunshine vitamin. Consequently, it's quite likely that supplementing with 2000 to 5000 IU of vitamin D-3 daily and Omega-3 fish oil will help substitute for our missed sun exposure when it comes to preventing seasonal mood swings.

Wearing bright yellow clothing works well for me in dealing with the lack of sunshine during the rainy Oregon winters. Studies associate yellow with: mental clarity, optimism, self esteem, and inspiration. This can improve mood, memory and concentration, and increase confidence, curiosity and courage. A bright yellow sweatshirt provides me with more, bang-for-the-buck, mood enhancement than any patented prescription is ever likely to. And there are no side-effects to wearing yellow.

Learning when to say "No" to your doctor can be a life saving skill. Drugs should always be your last choice and that is *never* more true than in the case of prescription anti-depressants.

15

Being An "Indoor Environmentalist"

Clean Doesn't Have A Smell

Whenever environmental pollution is mentioned, thoughts of polluted air and streams, electromagnetic pollution from high voltage power lines, and cell phone towers invariably come to mind. We seldom think about pollution being in the very place where we spend most of our time, inside of our own home. Considering that this is the only environment where we have almost total control, it may be worth our while to take a closer look.

Many people understand that when we remodel or update the inside of our homes, new paints, carpet, and other building materials can off-gas toxic

> If a product promises "April Freshness," an "Irish Spring" or "Sunshine and Fresh Mountain Air" in a box, be wary. If it sounds too ridiculous to be true, you can be sure it is and it's probably toxic too.

fumes. We generally undertake projects like that only once a decade or so, and we know that airing out affected rooms will usually take care of this temporary problem. What about the chemicals that we are in contact with on an everyday basis, from household cleaners, laundry soaps and personal grooming products.

It's well accepted that commercially prepared toilet and oven cleaners are usually highly corrosive, and inhaling their fumes can be extremely irritating to the eyes and respiratory tract. The package warnings are pretty clear and the feedback is often immediate.

However, due to the fact that clothing is in contact with our skin virtually all day, every day, laundry products deserve the closest of scrutiny for potentially toxic ingredients. Many people do not realize that our skin is very permeable and outside substances can quickly be absorbed directly through it into the bloodstream. From there, toxins are often stored in fatty tissue and critical organs like the liver, kidneys, reproductive organs, and brain. Removing stains and soil from clothes and replacing them with toxic detergent residues is not a good trade-off.

Sodium Lauryl Sulfate (SLS) is a surfactant, detergent, and emulsifier commonly used in concrete garage floor cleaners, engine degreasers, and thousands more industrial applications because it is a very inexpensive foaming agent. However, in some ways, SLS carries a very high price tag. 16,000 studies document its toxicity and hazards. SLS is contained in virtually all mainstream laundry detergents but is *not* required to be listed on the labels.

SLS is also found in approximately 90% of all shampoos, including some that are labeled "natural." SLS is considered by the Environmental Working Group (EWG) to be the most dangerous ingredient in personal care products.

SLS belongs to a group of ingredients known as penetration enhancers. Because it is such a potent degreaser (very handy when scrubbing a garage floor), it strips the protective oils (lipids) from your skin's surface, upsetting natural moisture regulation. In order to manage your hair and scalp after shampooing with SLS, conditioners and moisturizing treatments become necessary. Stripping the skin of its natural lipids in this way also decreases its resistance to penetration, thereby increasing absorption of drugs and toxins up to a hundred-fold. In addition, purely from the perspective of vanity or fashion, it can also impair your ability to grow hair.

According to the Environmental Working Group, research studies on Sodium Lauryl Sulfate have shown potential links to:

- ⅄ Irritation of eyes
- ⅄ Organ toxicity
- ⅄ Developmental/reproductive toxicity
- ⅄ Neurotoxicity, endocrine disruption, ecotoxicology, and cellular changes
- ⅄ Possible mutations and cancer

When is your home too clean? **Triclosan** is the bactericide used in most antibacterial soaps and other personal care products such as body washes, toothpastes, and deodorants. To further *protect* us (allegedly) from disease and infection it is often added into the manufacture of furniture, kitchenware, clothing, and toys.

Triclosan has now been linked to heart disease, heart failure, and hormonal disturbances. High levels of triclosan have been found to reduce sperm in male fish and cause them to develop female physical characteristics. It was first registered with the EPA in 1969 ... as a pesticide. Would you knowingly brush your teeth with pesticides or apply them to your underarms? Triclosan is clearly listed on product ingredient labels, so you can easily check to see if it's there before deciding on a purchase.

In addition, triclosan is building up in the environment. All those soaps and toothpastes go down the drain and eventually back into the water supply. A 2008 study, which was designed to assess exposure to triclosan in a representative sample of US children and adults, found it in the urine of nearly 75 percent of those tested. It has also been found in the umbilical cord blood of infants and in the breast milk of mothers.

A University of Minnesota study published in January 2013 in the journal *Environmental Science and Technology* said increasing amounts of triclosan were found in the sediment in eight Minnesota lakes and rivers. In 2014 Minnesota became the first state to ban triclosan in consumer products.

According to the FDA, there is no scientific evidence that triclosan provides any extra benefits to anyone's health beyond a marginal ability to reduce cavities, plaque, and inflammation when in toothpaste. Triclosan is currently under review by the FDA and Health Canada

Another very real contributor to in-home pollution dangers are **fabric softeners and dryer sheets.** Even though they may make your clothes feel soft and smell fake-fresh, fabric softeners and dryer sheets are some of the most toxic products used in the laundering process.

Fragrances added to many laundry products and other cleaners, may cause acute effects such as respiratory irritation, headache, sneezing, and watery eyes in sensitive individuals or allergy and asthma sufferers. The National Institute of Occupational Safety and Health has found that one-third of the substances used in the fragrance industry are toxic. But because the chemical formulas of fragrances are considered trade secrets, companies aren't required to list their ingredients but merely label them as: contains "fragrance."

When a product promises "April Freshness," an "Irish Spring," or "Sunshine and Fresh Mountain Air" in a box, be wary. **Remember: clean doesn't have a smell.** No matter what Tide, Cheer, or Clorox tells you, you can't package the environment for individual consumption - and if they could they'd be charging a lot more than $7.99 a box.

The cosmetics industry in the US totals nearly $50 billion in sales annually. The Food and Drug Administration (FDA), which "regulates" it, defines cosmetics as "intended to be applied to the human body for cleansing, beautifying, promoting attractiveness, or altering the appearance *without* affecting the body's structure or functions." From this, we may conclude that the FDA doesn't readily acknowledge that toxins from these products can easily pass through the skin. Consequently, in the FDA's view, no in-depth, long-term, safety testing on this class of products is required.

The bottom line is that cosmetics, including soaps and shampoos, are not considered foods or drugs, and are therefore are not subject to Food and Drug Administration approval

for long-term safety. Instead, the FDA allows the industry to self-monitor. So, the only systematic testing that is done is that which is done by manufacturers themselves or by the industry's trade group, the Cosmetic, Toiletry, and Fragrance Association. Research is reviewed by an industry-funded panel.

Environmental Working Group's (EWG) Vice President for Research, Jane Houlihan, says, "It's an anything-goes system. The companies making money off these products define what "safe" is. They define what it means to "substantiate" a product's safety."

You as a consumer have no way to know what safety testing - if any - is conducted on cosmetics containing known cancer triggers. Toxic exposure from products you might use daily can pose a serious health risk.

Healthy, Environmentally Sound Solutions

When gauging ecological claims of laundry and cleaning products, look for specifics. For example, "biodegradable in three to five days" holds a lot more meaning than "biodegradable," as most substances will eventually break down if given enough time and the right ecological conditions. For example, plastic bottles and bags can take 500 years or more, but they are technically "biodegradable." Also, statements like "no solvents," "no phosphates," or "plant-based" are more meaningful than vague terms like "ecologically-friendly" or "natural."

A few safe, simple ingredients like soap, water, baking soda, vinegar, lemon juice, and borax, aided by a little elbow grease and a coarse sponge for scrubbing, can take care of most household cleaning needs. They can also save you lots of money wasted on unnecessary specialized cleaners.

The Dr. Bronner's family has been making organic soaps for over 150 years and their liquid castile soaps diluted in water have hundreds of household uses. All of their scents come from organic essential oils. Dr. Bronner's* soaps are the *Swiss Army Knife* of the soap world – wash your dishes, your car, your bike, your hair, and even brush your teeth with them. Citra Solv, a concentrated, natural citrus based degreaser, is exceptionally effective and very economical when diluted in water. It's extremely versatile, with dozens of potential household uses - counter-tops, laundry (especially for grease stains), toilets, and even cleaning furniture and car seat fabrics (not leather).

We've all heard accounts of tough, 90 year old geezers with cast-iron constitutions who attribute their longevity to smoking a pack-a-day along with two or three shots of Scotch. On the other hand, we also hear stories of people who are so delicate and sensitive they practically get allergic reactions by just reading about a bad air quality day. The majority of us fall somewhere in between and would be wise to consciously avoid daily exposure to toxic chemicals that may cause damaging long-term health effects like cancer or hormonal imbalances, even if those effects are not immediately obvious.

---

* Dr Bronner's has been a major supporter of GMO labeling campaigns, donating millions of dollars to that cause. For that reason, combined with the fact that their soaps are great, they get my business.

16

Friends Don't Let Friends Drink Tap Water

Ensure Your Drinking And Bathing Water Is Safe

In the small southern Oregon town where I live a City Hall Newsletter mailed to all residents several years ago showed a picture depicting our city's smiling mayor supposedly enjoying a glass of city tap water, next to an article written that attempted to dispel fears about toxins in the water supply. Yet in the last five years at every City Committee, Commission, or Council meeting that I've attended, the only water offered to our City leaders has been bottled or filtered - never water straight from the City tap - why? Our illustrious, smiling mayor aside, the city leaders must know something the general public doesn't.

The Environmental Working Group (EWG) has once again released a report that deserves our attention. After analyzing water samples from 201 municipal water systems from 43 states, EWG found chemicals considered "probable human carcinogens" in every single water system they tested.

Before 1908, typhoid, cholera, and dysentery were real threats to populations drinking from municipal water systems. As a response, cities began using chlorine to disinfect water because it's very effective in preventing the spread of most diseases caused by water-borne pathogens.

However, no creature on the planet living in a natural environment has ever consumed chlorinated water. Chlorine is a poison that has many serious, adverse effects on human health. In the 1970s it was discovered that chlorinated water forms Trihalomethanes (THMs), or chlorine by-products, when the chlorine mixes with naturally occurring organic matter in groundwater supplies, like vegetation and algae. There is no debate that THMs are highly carcinogenic. The National Cancer Institute estimates total cancer rates to be up to 93% higher for people who consume chlorinated water than for people who do not. One published study showed an increase of 80% in bladder cancer rates alone, for those consuming chlorinated water.

In his book, Coronaries/Cholesterol/Chlorine, Joseph M. Price, MD presents startling evidence that THMs are the "prime causative agents of arteriosclerosis and its inevitable result, the heart attack or stroke." I've read the letter the EPA wrote to Dr. Price stating his work was extremely valuable and deserved further discussion. I've seen no evidence that the EPA ever publicly discussed this matter further.

Taking a hot, chlorinated, shower or bath may even be more dangerous than drinking it. More chlorine is absorbed directly through the skin and inhaled in the steam from one typical shower than is taken in from drinking five glasses of tap water. The heat and steam opens the pores allowing a high absorption of chlorine and other chemicals. Steam from a shower can contain 20 times the concentration of chlorine as tap water. Inhalation of chlorine vapors are a suspected cause of bronchitis and asthma. A report in the *American Journal of Public Health* links chlorine to increases not only of cancer, but skin irritations and asthma as well. It stated that "up to 2/3 of the harmful exposure to chlorine was due to skin absorption and inhalation from shower water." The US EPA recently wrote, "Due to chlorine and showering, virtually every home in America also has a detectable level of chloroform gas in the air." Chloroform was once a widely used anesthetic. Its vapor depresses the central nervous system and is also a strong respiratory irritant.

The good news is that chlorine and most other chemicals are easily removed from tap and shower water with a simple, inexpensive point-of-use (POU) water filter. Any filter is better than no filter, but models that meet or exceed NSF (formerly the National Sanitation Foundation) standards 42 and 53 are worth far more in health benefits than they cost. For home use, to make enough pure water to be convenient for drinking and cooking, you will want an under-counter or faucet mounted filter with continuous output as contrasted with a pour through pitcher design. In the shower a simple, screw-on, inline filter attaches between the water line and showerhead. POU filters for sinks are extremely valuable for bathing infants and bathtub filters are especially valuable for children and pregnant woman who enjoy a relaxing bath.

Top quality POU filters will provide safe drinking water for as little as about five cents per gallon. Due to the costs of replacement filters, units with the lowest initial purchase price will often cost significantly more in the long run than units with a higher initial purchase price, such as those that come with cartridges designed and certified to last 500 - 1500 gallons. The higher quality under-counter models can also be connected to a sink-mounted spigot, sink-mounted instant hot water heater, as well as your refrigerator's water and ice dispensers.

Unlike chlorine, water fluoridation (the practice of adding industrial-grade fluoride chemicals to water for the purpose of preventing tooth decay) isn't intended to treat the water, but to treat you, the person drinking the water. The FDA accepts that fluoride is a drug, not a nutrient, when used to prevent disease. By definition, therefore, fluoridating water is a form of medication. But is the public water supply an appropriate place to be adding drugs or health supplements? What's next at your faucet, vitamin-C and Valium?

The Oral Health Division of the Centers for Disease Control (CDC) hails fluoridation as one of the "top ten public health achievements of the 20th century." Yet comprehensive data from the World Health Organization reveals that there is no discernible difference in tooth decay between the minority of Western nations that fluoridate water, and the majority that do not. The US, which fluoridates over 70% of its water supplies, has more people drinking fluoridated water than the rest of the world combined. Most developed nations, including all of Japan and 97% of Western Europe, do not fluoridate their water.

Fact: fluoride is a highly toxic substance. That's why the FDA now requires a poison warning on all fluoride toothpastes sold in the US. A recently published Harvard University meta-analysis of 27 studies published over 22 years has concluded that children who live in areas with highly fluoridated water have "significantly lower IQ scores than those who live in low fluoride areas." Fluoride is also known to cause a cosmetically damaging effect called fluorosis, a staining of the teeth that has a significantly higher rate of occurrence if fluoride supplements (and fluoridated water) are used in the first six months of life.

If the political will in your city or state exists to remove or keep fluoridation out of the municipal supply, that's likely a far more realistic solution than filtering, because filtering fluoride involves an expensive and bulky reverse-osmosis filter that is simply unrealistic for the majority of people to buy.

The Fluoride Action Network website states: "As is becoming increasingly clear, fluoridating water supplies is an outdated, unnecessary, and dangerous relic from a 1950s public health culture that viewed mass distribution of chemicals much differently than many people do today."

In recent years, communities throughout the United States and Canada have started to reassess the conventional wisdom of fluoridating their water. Many of these communities, including over 50 since 2010, are reaching the obvious conclusion: when stripped of its endorsements, well-meaning intentions, and PR-praise, fluoridation of drinking water has no merit and may be dangerous.

How Much Do You Need To Drink?

Having established that pure water is the only healthy choice, the question becomes: How much of it do you need to drink? Growing up in the sixties, the single serving bottled water industry did not yet exist. Refillable, personal water bottles were equally foreign. Yet today, it's gotten to the point where most of us don't dare to take a walk around the block without wearing a camelBak hydration backpack or having a case of chilled designer sports drinks waiting for us the moment we arrive home so that our "recovery" from the walk goes smoothly. It may leave you wondering: Is proper hydration really as complex as "experts" make it sound?

Water definitely needs to be replenished often. You can exist for months without food, but only a few days without water. It is essential for survival. Blood, muscles, and lungs are all more than 75% water. Our brain is about 90% water and even bones are about 22% water.

Water helps regulate body temperature, lubricates and cushions joints, protects the spinal cord and other sensitive tissues, and gets rid of wastes through urination and perspiration. Water provides the means for transporting nutrients to our organs and tissues and helps to carry oxygen. Because we lose water every day through urine and sweat, taking in too little leads to dehydration.

Nonetheless, the concept of eight glasses of water, per day, for everyone regardless of size, environment, and activity level, is unfounded. Dr. Margaret McCartney, writing for the *British Medical Journal,* stated that the advice to drink eight glasses of water a day is "thoroughly debunked nonsense" being spread by bottled water companies in order to churn up more profit.

Writing in the *American Journal of Physiology,* Heinz Valtin of Dartmouth Medical School stated that, "there is no scientific data that comes close to verifying the need for everyone to be drinking eight glasses of water per day."

If you think about it, the one-size-fits-all concept of eight glasses per day is more than a little silly. Would it mean that a

110 lb. woman should drink as much as a 250 lb. man? Would it mean that no matter what your diet consists of, we should all drink the same amount? The obvious answer is no.

In truth, there is no one-size-fits-all answer for appropriate water intake. Proper hydration is dependent on a wide range of factors: the foods you eat, the climate you live in, your level of activity, as well as how much you, as an individual, perspire. The climate where I live is hot and dry all summer and cold and damp all winter. Accordingly, I drink about four to seven glasses of water per day in summer and three or four per day in winter. Outdoor exercise in summer can increase that for me by an additional three or four glasses daily. When your body loses one to two percent of its total water, your thirst mechanism kicks in to let you know it's time to drink. Thirst should be your guide. Drinking when you are mildly thirsty but not desperate for a drink will allow you to remain hydrated.

Fortunately, our bodies are designed with natural troubleshooting as well. A strong odor to your urine, along with a yellow or amber color, often indicates that you may be dehydrated. Studies show that healthy, well-hydrated people generally urinate about six to eight times per day. Symptoms of mild dehydration include thirst, muscle cramps, pains in joints, muscles, lower back aches, headaches, loss of energy, and constipation.

Dr. Joseph Mercola wrote: "As you age, your thirst mechanism tends to work less efficiently. Therefore, older adults will want to be sure to drink water regularly, in sufficient quantity to maintain pale yellow urine. As long as you aren't taking riboflavin (vitamin B2, found in most multivitamins), which turns urine bright "fluorescent" yellow, then your urine should be quite pale. If you have kidney or bladder stones or a urinary tract infection, increase your water intake accordingly."

In addition to drinking water, there are many ways for our bodies to take in water without directly drinking it. **Most fruits and vegetables consist of 85-95% water.** In contrast, a peanut butter sandwich probably measures less than 25% water, by weight. Therefore a person eating a lunch consisting of a large salad topped with some chicken, turkey, meat, or egg is probably getting more than triple the water of someone eating a peanut butter sandwich. The water needs of these two people would be drastically different.

People doing a lot of outdoor physical work in the heat or those exercising extremely hard may benefit from a sports drink that replenishes water and the electrolyte trace minerals lost in sweat. However, many sports drinks are expensive and unnecessarily high in sugars. Over time, the excess sugar will dehydrate you and deplete energy. A sudden burst of energy will be followed by a debilitating crash, as your pancreas and other glands do what they can to balance out the stimulation to your blood sugar.

Most sports drinks also contain processed salt, which, in theory, replenishes the electrolytes you lose while sweating. But, unless you're sweating profusely and for an extended period, the extra salt (especially of the highly refined variety) is unnecessary, and might be harmful.

The leading brands of sports drinks on the market typically contain as much as two-thirds the sugar of soda drinks and more sodium. They also often contain High-Fructose Corn Syrup (HFCS), artificial flavors, and food coloring, none of which belong in your body. In contrast; coconut water is one of nature's perfect sports drinks because it contains an excellent balance of electrolytes, tastes great, and is low in sugar.

If water isn't enough to keep you properly hydrated, try the following recipe for a homemade sports drink that will replenish fluids and electrolytes. It's inexpensive and good tasting. One of the key ingredients is a pinch of high quality sea salt which provides over 70 of the trace minerals lost in sweat.

- ⚓ 3 cups pure water
- ⚓ 1 cup organic fruit juice ... **OR**
- ⚓ an additional cup of water along with 1 Tablespoon of raw honey
- ⚓ 1/4 teaspoon of unrefined sea salt
- ⚓ Shake well before drinking.

If you know you will be exercising or doing heavy work in the heat the following day, you can drink up the day before. Pure, toxin-free water is the ideal beverage of choice for hydration, but remember you can get valuable fluids from fresh fruits and vegetables. The most highly refined dehydration monitor is thirst. You should drink when thirsty and on especially hot days, drink extra.

17

The Truth About
Non-Stick Cookware

Don't Be The Canary In Your Own Coal Mine

Even if you enjoy preparing healthy food you may be unknowingly poisoning yourself by using the wrong cookware. Pots and pans coated with Teflon, or any of the similar surfaces chemically analogous to Teflon, are immensely popular. US consumers spent approximately $1.2 billion on 159 million pots and pans last year, 60% of which were nonstick. But, **the health risks associated with common non-stick cookware greatly outweigh the small benefits to convenience.**

Although the technology has improved, the essential nonstick ingredient is the same as it was when a DuPont Company chemist discovered it in 1938. In 1954, a French inventor figured out a way to bond Teflon to frying pans and in 1960, the FDA approved using Teflon for cookware in the US. Teflon is the most well-known brand name for the chemical Perfluorooctanoic Acid (PFOA).

In June 2005, a scientific advisory panel to the US Environmental Protection Agency (EPA) identified PFOA (Teflon) as a "likely carcinogen" but drew no conclusions as to whether products made with it pose a cancer risk to humans. However, it did say that animal studies have identified four types of tumors in rats and mice exposed to PFOA. In 2008, 48 years after it was first approved, the EPA finally got around to issuing its final conclusion about PFOA (Teflon) and identified it as a human carcinogen.

In addition to being used to create non-stick cookware, PFOA is used to make many common products including the stain and grease repellent coatings for fast food containers, clothing, and carpeting (Scotchgard).

I still vividly remember the day in the early 60s when my family first used a Teflon frying pan. My brother and I shared our dad's amazement as we watched a fried egg slide effortlessly around an oil-free pan like a champion figure skater gliding gracefully over the ice. Little did we know, very negative health and environmental impacts of Teflon would later be discovered.

DuPont now acknowledges that Teflon coated cookware will break down and begin releasing carcinogenic fumes when heated to 446 degrees. They recommend keeping pot and pan temperatures below that. Trouble is, **after about five minutes of heating on a home stove, pans can easily reach temperatures of 680 degrees, or more, at which point Teflon releases at least six toxic gasses.** If your non-stick cookware reaches 1,000 degrees (unlikely in a home setting), a temperature that scientists have measured from stove top drip pans, the coatings will break down into a chemical warfare agent known as PFIB, very similar to the WWI "choking agent", phosgene gas. **I guess that means that as**

long as you keep your non-stick cookware away from your stove, you'll be perfectly safe.

The fumes from Teflon are known to kill birds, and cookware manufacturers actually warn against use of these pans in homes with pet birds. Guess what? Long term exposure to fumes that are toxic enough to kill your pet canary will, in large enough doses, probably kill you too!

Another problem is that once the non-stick surface has been overheated, it will degrade more easily the next time. The same is true if the cooking surface gets scratched or damaged.

For pollution related to the manufacture of Teflon, **DuPont recently paid out $107.6 million, settling a class-action suit and admitted that it hid medical data about the dangerous health effects of Teflon for 20 years**. They may have to pay up to $300 million in additional environmental fines. PFOA is currently found in the bloodstream of 95 percent of American men, women, and children

The Best and Safest Materials For Cookware

Enamel-Coated Cast Iron: Enamel is essentially a type of glass, making it inert and non-reactive. With proper care, good enamel-coated cookware will last a lifetime. Since the base is cast iron, this cookware has exceptionally good heat distribution and retention. The main drawbacks are that it's heavy, somewhat expensive and, while durable, can be broken if handled carelessly. Overall, this type of cookware is a great choice.

Ceramic: Is inert and non-reactive making it extremely safe and there's virtually no chance of damage or a melt down if it is ever accidentally boiled dry and overheated. Quality ceramic cookware can go from the refrigerator or freezer straight to the stove-top or oven. It provides good heat distribution and retention.

Glass: Glass is completely inert and affordable, but highly breakable and does not conduct heat evenly. Tea or coffee brewed in a glass pot using pure water, tastes cleaner and *noticeably* better than the same beverage brewed in a metal pot. When serious herbalists brew medicinal remedies, they will *always* use glass or ceramic cookware for its inherent purity.

Very Good Choices For Cookware

Stainless Steel: Stainless steel is the least reactive metal, and many people consider it the most versatile and affordable healthy cookware option. Take care to buy high quality stainless that is perfectly smooth with a high polish. Otherwise it will be more likely to stick and be difficult to clean. The best stainless steel cookware will be laminated to an aluminum or cast iron outer bottom layer. This provides a clean, safe, non-reactive cooking surface on the inside and offers the even heat distribution of cast iron or aluminum on the outside.

Back in 1981, my brother and I were on a very limited budget and bought a restaurant full of used equipment at a substantial discount to start our first natural foods restaurant. A six-gallon aluminum soup pot was part of the deal. A replacement thick bottom, stainless steel soup pot of that size was beyond our means at that time. About once a week we simmered a batch of tomato sauce in the aluminum pot. Early on, we made a little profit and invested about $200 on a beautiful stainless steel pot to replace the aluminum one. I cooked the first batch of sauce in the new pot using our original recipe. Not knowing that the sauce had been made in the new pot, upon tasting it my brother asked: What did you change in the recipe?" He said that it tasted sweeter, fresher, and cleaner. Amazingly, the only change had been the new stainless steel pot – lesson learned.

Cast Iron: Cast iron is extremely durable, versatile and inexpensive. It features superior heat distribution and retention. When properly sealed (seasoned), cast iron cookware resists sticking. It requires consistent maintenance, but should last for generations.

Cookware To Avoid

Common non-stick or aluminum should be avoided. Aluminum is a soft, highly reactive metal that can leach into food, especially when you are cooking with acidic ingredients like tomatoes, vinegar, or lemon juice. The long-term health risks associated with these materials make them very poor choices. Copper interior cooking surfaces should also be avoided.

If you still have non-stick cookware in your home, it would be smart to invest in healthier alternatives. Considering that it's something you probably use almost daily, and that it should last decades, you'll be making a great, cost-effective, long-term investment in your health.

18

Frequent Cell Phone Use Can
Be Bad For Your Health

So Far, "Cigarette-Science" Claims
Cell Phones Are Perfectly Safe

There are now over 2 billion users of cell phones worldwide; 270 million of those subscribers are in the United States. And yet, startlingly, the question of cell phone safety has yet to be appropriately addressed by our government or manufacturers. Apple Inc. suggests users of their iPhones allow a minimum of 5/8 of an inch away from their bodies' to limit harmful radiation. **This seemingly vital piece of information regarding the safety of their top-selling device doesn't appear on the phone, or even the box** – but is buried in its owners' manual between sections on proper storage temperature and hearing aid compatibility. Further obscuring the truth, most of these phones no longer come with printed operating manuals. You actually have search for the information online.

If users can locate a manual and make it through the fine print, they would read that cell phones expose us to a form of electromagnetic radiation called radio frequency (RF) energy. Scientists have long thought that this radiation may increase the risk of brain cell damage that can, and does, lead to tumors (in 1995 they found this to be the case in laboratory experiments). Since then, the science behind cell phone danger has been suspiciously murky. Many neutral scientists have come to conclusions that would implicate cell phones as a major cause of brain cell damage and cancer – though other studies, which can be tied to corporations with a vested interest in telecommunications, have claimed no correlation – showing an eerie similarity of scruples to cigarette industry science.

Meanwhile, government agencies, have essentially ignored safety warnings by doctors and scientists; completely failing to acknowledge published research demonstrating that it can take between 10 to 30 years for brain tumors to develop from cell phone exposure. But decades-long lag time doesn't remove the very real dangers of cell phones. In fact, the abstract nature of cell phone dangers should put an even bigger onus on government to make their dangers known.

This isn't the first time US government officials have conveniently looked the other way instead of carefully scrutinizing a profitable new technology to protect a trusting public. The first documented death due to asbestos was in 1906. Asbestos-related diseases began to be commonly diagnosed in the 1920s but related workman's compensation cases were settled in secrecy for the next five decades. Well into the 1970s, asbestos was still used in a variety of construction applications. Later in the 70s, court documents proved that asbestos industry officials had worked hard to conceal the truth about asbestos toxicity from the unsuspecting public. Now it's scientifically accepted (and common knowledge) that Mesothelioma (a deadly cancer) is caused by exposure to asbestos.

The cell phone industry began in the early 1980s, when technologies developed for the Department of Defense were commercialized by telecommunication companies with an eye on profits. **Together, these groups lobbied to allow cell phones to be sold without pre-market safety testing**. They were successful, and the fledgling cell phone industry was exempted from regulatory oversight when it was most needed.

There is now a growing list of doctors, scientists, and consumer advocates who are drawing parallels between the blind faith of cell phone use in this century to the widespread acceptance of cigarettes as safe, in the 20th century. Certainly there are some clear parallels to be drawn between cell phones and cigarettes. Dr. Joseph Mercola has publicly pointed out where cell phones and cigarettes intersect:

- Manufacturers and industry insiders who either hide or attempt to debunk unfavorable study results and continue to promote their products despite awareness of the significant dangers to public health.
- Government conflict of interest created by lobbies for both industries and revenues collected from use taxes.
- Expensive, effective marketing campaigns aimed at every segment of society, including children.
- Massive amounts of scientific data proving beyond a shadow of a doubt the direct link between these products and life-threatening damage to the human body.
- The addictive nature of both products.

It appears as if the cell phone industry is fully aware of the dangers. In fact, some companies' service contracts prohibit suing the cell phone manufacturer or service provider, or joining a class action lawsuit. This indicates to me the likelihood that their lawyers know that enough scientific evidence exists about cell phone health hazards that they don't want to have to fight un-winnable cases in court. Still, the public is largely ignorant of the dangers, while the media regularly trumpet new studies showing cell phones are completely safe to use.

Despite denials from most in the cell phone industry, history may be repeating itself. More studies are released every year that implicate cell phone use with increases of:

- ⚔ Brain and head tumors
- ⚔ Visual problems
- ⚔ Sleep and memory disorders
- ⚔ Leukemia and more

Findings released in 2014 by researchers at Bordeaux University (France), supported other international studies, suggesting a higher threat of a brain tumors observed among heavier cell phone users. Using a cellphone for more than half an hour a day over five years can triple the risk of developing certain types of brain cancer, the French study suggests. Researchers found that people who used cell phones for 15 hours per month, on average, had a two to three times greater risk of developing glioma and meningioma - the main types of brain tumor - compared with those who used their phone rarely.

In 2008, cell phones were identified as a contributor to salivary gland tumors. Dr. Siegal Sadetzki, who testified in September 2009 at the US Senate Hearing, is the principle investigator of the study that made this finding: "Your risk of getting a parotid tumor on the same side of your head that you use for listening to the mobile phone increases by 34 to 58% depending on how frequently you use a cell phone."

According to the New York Times, "The largest study of cell phone use and brain cancer has been the Interphone International Case Control Study. The authors included disturbing data showing that **subjects who used a cell phone 10 or more years doubled the risk of developing brain gliomas, a type of tumor.**"

Using a cell phone pressed right up against your head immediately before going to bed (especially for a long call), can cause insomnia and may also cut your amount of deep sleep, interfering with your body's ability to refresh, rebuild, and repair itself.

The risks posed to children may be the most alarming of all. Because children's skulls are less dense and more easily penetrated by radio frequency radiation, children and adolescents are especially susceptible to the ill-effects of cell phone use. The Vienna Medical Association is demanding the banning of cell phone advertising targeting children and adolescents, advising against children under the age of 16 even using cell phones.

Cell phone technologies are clearly a case where we should be guided by the Precautionary Principle: an idea that suggests evidence of *probable* harm, rather than definitive *proof* of harm, should be all that is needed to shift the burden of proof from the innocent and often unsuspecting public to the producer of a potential public health risk.

Steps You Can Take To Reduce The Harmful Effects Of Cell Phone Use:

Keep them away from your head - Apple Inc. says your iPhone should come no closer than 5/8 of an inch; BlackBerry Ltd. recommends about an inch.

If you must use them near your head – switching ears occasionally (from left to right and back again) will reduce the chances of health complications.

Use the cell phone in speaker-phone mode - reduce close-proximity exposure to your head.

Turn your phone off whenever feasible - if possible, keep phones away from your body when they are on, by not attaching them to belts or carrying them in pockets.

Don't Chat with a Poor Signal - your phone emits more radiation when it has to work harder to find a signal.

Keep Your Phone Out of Your Pocket - a study published in the *Journal of Craniofacial Surgery* linked cell phone radiation to decreased bone density in the pelvis, and a 2008 study conducted by the Cleveland Clinic found that it lowers fertility in men.

Use your land-line home phone - remember those? Save long conversations for your home phone.

Consider texting rather than talking - not just for teenagers! Texting eliminates some of cell phones most harmful effects by keeping phone away from your head.

Given the track record that the government has protecting consumers, shouldn't we err on the side being safer now, rather than being sorry later? Despite their convenience, cell phones may affect multiple facets of your brain function, sleep patterns, and overall health. The ubiquity of cell phones doesn't equate to safety. In fact, as we've often seen, the ease of use and convenience of new technologies can create a false sense of safety. It's becoming alarmingly clear that the costs of cell phone ownership may be far greater than what appears on the bottom line of your monthly bill.

19

Sunshine Is Really Good

It's The Artificial Sunscreen That's Killing You

We've all been warned that sun exposure can cause skin cancer, but that's only a small part of the story. **The fact is that skin cancer was very rare 100 years ago and is still extremely rare among many populations who spend all day in the sun.** Statistically, the greatest rise in skin cancer has been in countries where chemical sunscreens have been heavily promoted. There is almost no skin cancer among dark skinned people living in Africa, while African-Americans have far higher rates of skin cancer and stay in the sun less than those in Africa.

It seems likely that the recent rise in skin cancers is due to factors other than just sun exposure. Drs. Cedric and Frank Garland of the University of California, San Diego, have pointed out that while sunscreens protect against sunburn, there is no scientific proof that they protect against melanoma or basal cell carcinoma in humans. Further, the Garlands believe that the increased use

153

of chemical sunscreens is the primary cause of the skin cancer epidemic. Dr. Marianne Berwick epidemiologist of Sloan Kettering Cancer Center, concluded after years of study that: "We don't really know if sunscreens prevent skin cancer at all."

Fact: many popular chemical sunscreens contain ingredients very likely to cause cancer. There are 17 individual sunscreen ingredients that are FDA approved. Fifteen are clear chemicals that absorb UV light. Of these, nine are known endocrine disruptors that interfere with the normal function of hormones. Two are made of minerals that reflect UV light.

Since the skin is a porous organ, chemical sunscreens don't just sit on the surface of the skin, they are absorbed into it and quickly find their way into the bloodstream. These chemicals reach all organs and tissues of the body before being detoxified by the liver. They have been found in breast milk, blood, and urine for up to two days after a *single* application. Since these chemicals cannot be considered safe, it is a problem. Because some sunscreens lose as much as 90% of their sun-blocking effectiveness in just an hour and need to be reapplied often, this can quickly become a major problem.

Most chemical sunscreens contain oxybenzone, a synthetic estrogen that easily penetrates the skin and contaminates the body. Oxybenzone and other endocrine disruptors can mimic real estrogen, feminize tissues and throw the body's systems out of balance. Oxybenzone can cause reproductive disorders in men and women and increase incidence of many different kinds of cancers, birth defects and innumerable other serious health problems.

Over 40% of sunscreens contain topical vitamin A, often listed as retinyl palmitate. Recent government studies have shown that tumors and lesions develop 21% faster when skin coated with vitamin A is exposed to sunlight. Slathering up before heading outside on a sunny day doesn't sound like the smartest option.

The effects of acute toxins are easy to recognize and become obvious quickly after exposure. Poisoning that takes place slowly over decades is very difficult to pinpoint and study reliably. **Rather than humans being the long-term guinea pigs in this experiment, the FDA needs to step up and do the science now.**

The Food and Drug Administration's 2007 sunscreen safety regulations state: "FDA is not aware of data demonstrating that sunscreen use alone helps prevent skin cancer." The International Agency for Research on Cancer (IARC) agrees and recommends clothing, hats, and shade as primary barriers to UV radiation stating that "sunscreens should not be the first choice for skin cancer prevention and should not be used as the sole agent for protection against the sun."

It is problematic that for decades conventional Western doctors and cosmetic companies have strongly advocated liberal application of chemical sunscreens before any exposure to sunlight, even for young children. This is despite the fact that there has never been adequate safety testing of the primary chemicals in these products or sufficient discussion questioning the need for sunscreens at all.

Is Sunscreen Really Necessary?

The answer is: maybe ... sometimes. For instance, if you live in a Northern climate and take a sun-filled winter vacation, your body would not have adequate time during a short vacation to gradually tan and build up thicker skin. Or if you have an indoor job and plan to spend the first sunny weekend of the summer outside it would be best to use a safe, natural sunscreen because they help prevent sunburn and its accompanying skin damage. If you have time to gradually increase your sun exposure, sunscreen may not be necessary or advisable.

Sunscreens definitely reduce vitamin D production and as a result reduce the numerous powerful health benefits natural, sun-created vitamin D provides, including cancer prevention. Exposure to sunlight has also recently been proven to help reduce blood pressure. It is likely that using sunscreen will diminish that effect.

Alternatives to Sunscreen:

Wear clothes - shirts, hats, shorts, and pants shield your skin from the sun's UV rays – and don't coat your skin with goop. Early in the season a light-weight long-sleeved shirt is a good start.

Find shade – or make it - picnic under a tree, read beneath an umbrella, take a canopy to the beach. Keep infants in the shade – they lack tanning pigments (melanin) to protect their skin.

Plan around the sun - if your schedule is flexible, go outdoors in early morning or late afternoon when the sun is lower in the sky. UV (ultraviolet) radiation peaks at midday, when the sun is directly overhead.

Don't get burned - red, sore, blistered (then peeling) skin is a clear sign you've gotten far too much sun. Repeated sunburn increases skin cancer risk. Once the skin turns pink the health benefits of vitamin D production cease.

When choosing sunscreens you'd be smart to completely avoid those with vitamin A (retinol or retinyl palmitate), and oxybenzone. Far safer active ingredients are zinc oxide or titanium dioxide (basically ground rocks that reflect sunlight). Inactive, skin nourishing organic ingredients could include coconut oil, jojoba oil, vitamins D and E, sunflower oil, or shea butter. Choose a sunscreen effective against UVA and UVB radiation. A word of caution – I've found that one formula from a given manufacturer may be safe while another from the *same* company may have dangerous ingredients. Do your homework or shop at a health food store that does the research for you. Then go out for some warm weather fun in the sun.

Benefits of Sun Exposure

Dr. Robert S. Stern, chair of the Department of Dermatology at Harvard-affiliated Beth Israel Deaconess Medical Center, calls people so concerned about getting skin cancer that they stay inside or cover every bit of skin "solar-phobes." Nobody wants to get skin cancer, but we've gone from sun worship to sun dread.

Many of the sun's benefits are so fundamental, they're often overlooked, even taken for granted. But direct sun exposure is a major ingredient of the conditions that humans evolved with. Our bodies' functions aren't just made easier by the sun, they're directly catalyzed by it. **Removing, or greatly reducing**

sun exposure from your daily life is to rob yourself of the condition under which you are designed to thrive. At the most fundamental levels, the sun synchronizes important biorhythms via the sunlight entering your eye, striking your retina and reaching your brain through the optic nerve. The sun regulates body temperature, as well as enhances mood and energy through the release of endorphins.

The sun's list of benefits extends much further than the more basic facilitation of your body's biorhythms, and though they may seem less intuitive at face value, have been proven through billions of years of life on earth, as well as the scientific method. That list includes treating skin diseases, such as psoriasis, vitiligo, atopic dermatitis, and scleroderma. The sun's UV radiation also enhances skin barrier functions, relieves fibromyalgia pain, and protects against and suppresses symptoms of multiple sclerosis (MS). The standard treatment for tuberculosis 100 years ago, long before the advent of antibiotics was nothing more than direct sun exposure.

In a recently released landmark study, the researchers at the University of Edinburgh in the United Kingdom found that when sunlight touches our skin, a compound called nitric oxide that helps lower blood pressure, is released into our blood vessels. Nitric oxide also helps protect your skin against UV damage and promotes wound healing through its antimicrobial effect. These are but a few common benefits of the sun. You could argue, save for a few very rare exceptions, that adding a moderate amount of sun exposure is the perfect companion to your existing methods of treatment.

Richard Weller, Senior Lecturer in Dermatology, says the effect is such that overall, sun exposure could improve health and even prolong life, because the benefits of reducing blood pressure, cutting heart attacks and strokes and balancing the endocrine system far outweigh the small likelihood of increased risk of getting skin cancer.

Plus ...the sun feels soooo good.

20

Cancer Patients Have Many New Options

Integrative Medicine Treats Patients As Individuals

In the past 35 years, I've seen virtually every cancer healing modality work* - and seen all of them fail. That includes prayer, fasting, detoxification, special diets, vitamin therapy, surgery, radiation, and chemotherapy. **The most appropriate question becomes: which method, or combination of methods, are best for an *individual* person's circumstances?**

When I am asked, "what's the best cancer treatment?" **the advice I usually offer is for people to thoroughly research the available options and then choose the ones that *they* personally feel most confident about.** Ultimately - beyond just surviving the disease - I believe that having confidence in the totality of their treatment will provide people the best chance for a strong, healthy, post cancer-diagnosis life.

Today, the use of synthetic drugs and surgery to treat health conditions is known simply as "conventional medicine." This is the kind of medicine most Americans still encounter in hospitals and clinics. Often both expensive and invasive, it is also very good at some things - for example, handling emergency conditions such as massive injury or immediate survival after a life-threatening heart attack or stroke. However, **for long-term care of a chronic condition, there are almost always much better options than conventional medicine (see chapter three).**

A well respected, forward thinking physician in my area (southern Oregon), Dr. Robin Miller, recently published an article that offered excellent, common sense, affordable advice on maintaining health and preventing breast cancer. Her well-documented piece includes information about the highly beneficial roles that exercise, vitamin D, flaxseed, medicinal mushrooms, and cruciferous vegetables can play in breast cancer prevention *and* treatment.

Unfortunately, most patients in southern Oregon do not hear this kind of advice from their own doctor. I know this because people frequently come into our health food store confused by the lack of serious consideration their doctors give to diet, nutrition, exercise, and holistic health approaches in general. If the typical MD says anything about natural cancer treatment modalities, it's likely to be something like: "So as long as you're doing chemo, radiation, drugs, and surgeries – you might as well throw in the natural stuff too." Not exactly a confidence-inspiring endorsement of a holistic approach to healing.

Following the money may provide a better understanding of the typical doctor's lack of enthusiasm for natural, time-tested practices. Doctors, such as oncologists, anesthesiologists, radiologists, and cardiologists, who typically specialize in treating acute, life-threatening conditions using drugs and surgeries, receive an average annual income of approximately $300,000. The average annual income for a member of the American College of Preventative Medicine, a group of preventative medical doctors, is $100,000. When it comes to publicity from the news or entertainment media, dramatic medical interventions sell. Without ever watching a single episode, you can be sure that a TV show named E.R. (emergency room - featuring crisis, action, speed, EKG flat-lines and shocking paddles) would easily win the ratings war with a show called P.M. (preventative medicine - where physically fit patients would casually walk in, breathe deeply, smile, and listen to calming music while enjoying a cup of herbal tea in the waiting room).

At one time, all medicine was natural and revolved around medicinal plants, natural rhythms, and most importantly, a close observation by a healer of the whole person. Hippocrates, the ancient Greek physician, is often regarded as the "Father of Western Medicine" and credited with the quote: "let food be thy medicine." He believed in the healing power of nature and the power of our bodies to heal themselves. But as medicine that depends on expensive drugs and surgery became the *new normal*, age-old wisdom was forced into the background. **In their cancer-fighting toolbox, most oncologists today have tools that address the disease in only one of three ways – cut, burn, or poison.**

Though progress is slow, there's an increasing constituency of doctors and patients who are bonding with the philosophy of Integrative Medicine (IM) and its whole-person approach. An approach designed to treat the person, not just the disease. IM depends on a partnership between the patient and the doctor, where the goal is to treat body, mind, and spirit. While some of the therapies used may be non-conventional, a guiding principle within Integrative Medicine is to primarily rely on therapies that have a reasonable amount of high-quality evidence to support them.

In his *New York Times* review of Dr. Andrew Weil's (Integrative Medicine's most prominent practitioner), latest book, <u>Healthy Aging: A Lifelong Guide to Your Physical and Spiritual Well-Being</u>, Abraham Verghese, MD, summed up this orientation well, stating that Dr. Weil "doesn't seem wedded to a particular dogma, Western or Eastern, only to **the get-the-patient-better philosophy."**

In contrast, the national health and cancer care debates are usually dominated by financial concerns rather than "getting the patient well." Dr. Peter Glidden, noted author and naturopathic physician, who regularly treats cancer patients using more holistic approaches stated: **"The primary reason chemotherapeutic methods are usually employed to treat to cancer is because they are highly profitable."**

Dr. Ralph Moss has studied cancer treatments for five decades and written eight books, including his most recent work, <u>Cancer Therapy: The Independent Consumer's Guide to Non-Toxic Treatment.</u> He also wrote <u>The Cancer Industry,</u> a documented research work telling of the enormous financial and political corruption in the "cancer establishment." He believes that the motivating forces in cancer research and treatment are often power and money and not the cure of cancer patients. However, Moss is very fair. He acknowledges that chemotherapy is often effective for about 2% to 4% of specific types of cancer, but in 96% to 98% of cancers chemo is basically useless. Moss says that the vast majority of cancers, such as breast, colon, and lung cancer are barely touched by chemotherapy.

As defined by the FDA, the words "effective cancer treatment," become a matter of semantics. The FDA defines an "effective" drug as one which achieves a 50% or more reduction in tumor size for 28 days. According to Moss, in the vast majority of cases there is absolutely no correlation between shrinking tumors for 28 days and the cure of the cancer or extension of patient life.

Further, Integrative Health practitioner Dr. Nicholas Gonzales states: "There is so much collusion between government research institutions like the NCI (National Cancer Institute) and the drug companies. I know because I worked with the NCI for ten years and it's like a business school for the drug industry! There are a thousand full-time drug company lobbyists in Washington. That's two for every congressman and senator! They are all working full-time, making six figure incomes and trying to influence medical legislation."

Their conclusions are supported by the results of a five-year study conducted by the Department of Radiation Oncology, Northern Sydney Cancer Centre in Australia. That study showed that even though chemotherapy is extremely expensive (especially in the US) and can have severe side-effects, it only improved five-year cancer survival rates in the US by 2.1%. It's likely that extreme amounts of money, effort, and time **(and for cancer patients *time* is often the most valuable resource)** could be better utilized with methodologies that produce far more patient improvement per dollars and days invested.

Of the twelve drugs approved by the Food and Drug Administration in 2012 for various cancer conditions, eleven were priced above $100,000 for a year of treatment.

Why are cancer fighting drugs so expensive? One reason is that the US pharmaceutical industry spent 24.4 percent of each dollar of sales on promoting the drugs, as compared to 13.4 percent spent on research and development, according to a 2008 study in *PLOS* Medicine by York University researchers who collected data from the pharmaceutical industry and physicians. **However, the discussion about drug prices and people's ability to pay them really only distracts from the much bigger issue, which is the true value (or lack of value) of the drugs themselves.**

Big Pharma loves the new US healthcare program because virtually all of their products will all be covered by the new health insurance laws. Drug companies will continue to make billions selling toxic medications that often offer little actual improvement. There is nothing in the new legislation that favors Integrative Medicine. Integrative Medicine recognizes that conventional and natural approaches can be used separately with success, but together, may often create better patient outcomes.

Treating Patients As Unique Individuals Greatly Increases Chances Of Success

An excellent example of a creative breakthrough for treating cancer is routinely used at Dr. Stanislaw Burzynki's medical clinic in Houston, TX. His customized gene therapies are tightly targeted to each patient's specific cancer. Dr. Burzynski is very experienced and has treated over 15,000 cancer patients. His medications attack a particular genetic feature, protein, or enzyme, unique to an individual patient's cancer.

Dr. Burzynski battled the FDA in court for over a decade for the right to offer his options to cancer patients. They basically tried to throw him in jail. The FDA monitors his claims and results very closely. Results from his clinic are good, especially considering that patients seeking his advice usually have advanced stage three or stage four cancers, and have already tried standard chemo and/or radiation treatments that have failed to improve their condition.

According to Burzynski, the problem with conventional oncology is that: "most oncologists work like robots. They give all of their patients the same treatment, but every patient is unique and has different needs. Oncologists have been trained to believe that radiation, chemotherapy, and surgery are the only ways to treat cancer. If they realized there is another universe out there consisting of treatments that work on the genes, they might want to do them, but most of them don't even think much about these alternative treatments."

Dr. Robert Zieve, an MD from Prescott, AZ, is one of the most experienced and well-trained physicians in integrative medicine in the US. He has practiced holistic and Integrative Medicine for 35 years and now focuses on treating patients with cancer. Zieve stated: "Thousands of published reports demonstrate the beneficial effects of herbs and nutrients upon cancer. I am hoping that more doctors will recognize their benefits, but until they do, one of the main messages that I impart to my patients is that they should interview their physicians. A one-size-fits-all approach to medicine doesn't work, and it's important for patients to put together their own team of competent practitioners who can help them to get better."

"We have had many patients who were supposed to die but who instead returned to their oncologists alive and thriving. When this happens, most oncologists don't ask their patients what they did to get well, and they don't explore their situations more. An attitude of inquiry should be present in a scientific mind, but in general, it's very lacking in modern oncology and modern medicine."

Burzynski's and Zieve's views on cancer are contained within the 2011 book, Defeat Cancer, by Connie Strasheim. It contains over 400 pages of interviews with 15 highly regarded Integrative Medicine practitioners who treat cancer and are dedicated to their patients' well-being, not to merely following drug company created protocols. It's probably the best single resource I know of on this subject. Interesting to note is that several of the Integrative Medicine practitioners featured in the book often recommend treating some kinds of testicular or blood cancers with chemo because for those *specific* cancers, chemo appears to provide positive results.

Further, many of the Integrative Medicine practitioners interviewed in Defeat Cancer offer unique techniques (IPT - Insulin Potentiation Therapy for example) that can optimize results using lower doses of chemo while minimizing unwanted side-effects. Patients of practitioners trained and experienced in using herbs, acupuncture, and optimization of nutrition often make it through chemotherapy protocols with minimal discomfort and their vitality (life force) largely intact. Holistically building patients' strength prior to administering chemo and working to minimize its undesirable side-effects are areas where Integrative practitioners offer approaches far superior to virtually anything offered by most mainstream oncologists.

The best way to use <u>Defeat Cancer</u> is to read it carefully and decide if any of the doctors featured offer treatments and embrace attitudes that make sense to you. If so, select the ones whose attitudes and advice resonates most with your gut feeling, then call or visit them. Choose those that you feel most confident about and then enthusiastically follow their advice.

Principles of Integrative Medicine:

⅄ A partnership between patient and practitioner in the healing process

⅄ Appropriate use of conventional and alternative methods to facilitate the body's innate healing response

⅄ Consideration of all factors that influence health, wellness, and disease including mind, spirit, and community, as well as body

⅄ A philosophy that neither rejects conventional medicine nor accepts alternative therapies uncritically

⅄ Recognition that good medicine should be based in good science, be inquiry driven, and be open to new paradigms

⅄ Use of natural, effective, less-invasive interventions whenever possible

⅄ Use of the broader concepts of promotion of health and the prevention of illness as well as the treatment of disease

⅄ Training of practitioners to be models of health and healing, committed to the process of self-exploration and self-development

There are many more cancer treatment options available than most patients will ever hear about from their oncologist. Patients need to be proactive and do some research to make the most informed choices possible when selecting their treatments. The relatively new field of Integrative Medicine is giving patients dozens of effective options to treat disease that conventional toxic medicines, when applied in conventional ways, have shown poor success rates for. This is reason for hope for many who desire alternatives.

Whatever cancer healing methods patients choose, it is vitally important that after doing their due-diligence, they move forward with confidence that they've chosen the treatments that *they* believe will give them the best chance to regain their health.

* Unforgettable Cancer Remission Story

I am relaying the following cancer healing anecdote only to share one woman's story and the possibilities it represents – not as an example of anything I think is common, or as a one-size-fits-all approach.

About 20 years ago, a woman (mother of one) in her mid-forties was a regular customer whom I knew to be a cancer survivor. However, the word survivor doesn't come close to describing her beautiful spirit; more than a survivor, she was a thriver. She was always very positive, grateful and forward thinking. One day, after knowing her for awhile, I asked her the details of her experiences with cancer. She was happy to share the following:

At some point she had been diagnosed with lung cancer, and after other conventional treatments had failed, she had a lung removed. About a year later doctors discovered more cancer and she was again scheduled for surgery.

This was years before many of today's advanced imaging and diagnostic tools were widely available. When the doctors opened her up, they realized the extent of the cancer, closed her back up and said that the cancer had advanced beyond the point where they could hope to help her condition.

She told me that, after consulting with her family, she decided to forgo using any more conventional remedies and instead began following a very specific natural diet, just so she could "die a more peaceful and less painful death."

She then said: "After about two or three months of following the diet, my husband looked in my eyes and said that he thought I was getting better." Then she asked: "Do you know when that was?" Of course I had no idea. She said: "that was 16 years ago!"

I will never forget her husband and daughter listening in silence as she shared her awe-inspiring story.

21

Natural Dietary Supplements Are Superior To Synthetic

Don't Be Misled By Research Controlled By Big Pharma and Mainstream Medicine

Good and thorough science adds clarity to any discussion. However, junk science is often very misleading. In 2013, the Fred Hutchinson Cancer Research Center in Seattle made a major contribution to junk science when it published the findings of their Selenium and vitamin E Cancer Prevention Trial (SELECT), claiming that Omega-3 fatty acids, the kind found in fish oil, increased prostate cancer risk. They also stated that taking vitamin E increases prostate cancer risk. Lead (so-called) researcher Alan Kristal stated: "We've shown once again that use of nutritional supplements may be harmful."

However, there are two big problems with their conclusions. Incredibly, no data was presented confirming that the men studied actually took fish oil supplements or even ate any fish. Further, the vitamin E studied was the totally synthetic D-L form. The D-L form is readily available at Wal-Mart and Rite Aid and in mass-market multivitamins but would never be sold at any reputable health food store. The slipshod methodology and faulty conclusions reached in this study are an insult to truth-seeking scientists everywhere.

While the study's authors offered the sweeping generalization that taking supplements may be harmful, they completely failed to acknowledge that the synthetic supplements they studied are vastly different than herbs and other natural supplements derived from organic and other non-GMO sources.

> Synthetic vitamins may be good for giving uninformed people a false sense of security, but they do nearly nothing to biologically improve your health.

Unfounded, sweeping generalizations aside, looking at dietary supplements with a broad view, **we find that herbal medicine supplementation goes back thousands of years, having been a part of virtually every civilization in history.** Unfortunately, herbalism in North America was set back several hundred years when European settlers killed and marginalized the Native American populations who embodied centuries of wisdom about the plants and herbs indigenous to this continent. In the last few decades we've begun to catch up thanks, in part, to the contributions of internationally respected American herbalists like: James Duke, Dr. John Christopher, and Ed Smith, co-founder of Herb Pharm.

I will say first, that it's best to get your vitamins from whole food sources because they provide complete vitamins rather **than** fractions of them. Common sense tells us that our bodies were designed to receive nutrition from the foods we eat. Raw, whole foods typically have the complementary enzymes, trace minerals, and co-factors our bodies need to readily assimilate all the nutrients. For example, sunflower seeds are an excellent natural source of vitamin E and the mineral selenium, both of which need the other to offer their full health and antioxidant benefits. However, short-sighted, profit-driven agricultural practices dating back to the 1930s have robbed the soil and therefore our food supply of sufficient amounts of many key nutrients. This problem has been 75 years in the making. A US Senate report written, amazingly, back in 1936 stated: "The alarming fact is that foods are now being raised on millions of acres of land that no longer contains enough of certain needed minerals. These foods are starving us - no matter how much we eat!"

Because most of our foods are processed and the overwhelming majority are not organic and grown in weak, exhausted soils, it may be virtually impossible today to achieve complete and balanced nutrition without some form of dietary supplementation. Further, the vast majority of meats today are derived from animals that are (unnaturally) fed grains rather than grazing on grasses in open pasture land. The fat profile in the meat from grain-fed cattle is significantly different and less healthy than the fat profile from grass-fed animals.

Livestock raised in non-traditional (unnatural) ways, inescapably produces meat, milk, and eggs with altered and diminished nutrient content. This creates the need for dietary supplementation and has largely contributed to the surge in popularity of Omega-3 fish oil supplements.

Unlike high quality, food-derived supplements, cheap multivitamins like Centrum (owned by drug industry giant, Pfizer pharmaceuticals), or One-A-Day (owned by Bayer, aspirin and GMO manufacturer) are nearly 100% synthetic. Synthetic nutrients have no direct biological link to anything that has ever lived on earth. Unless you were seriously ill from a deficiency disease, you would likely be better off not taking these synthetic imitations of nourishment. Centrum and One-A-Day also contain artificial colors and coatings. Their packaging and marketing probably cost more than the cheap raw materials inside the bottles. Nonetheless, Centrum generates about one billion dollars in sales annually for Pfizer. **Synthetic vitamins may be good for giving uninformed people a false sense of security, but they do nearly nothing to biologically improve your health and may even be harmful.** Eating carrots is good for you. Eating a plastic model of a carrot is not.

Fortunately, there are a growing number of ethical companies that produce top quality nutritional supplements that your body can truly benefit from. Garden of Life and New Chapter are two such vitamin companies. They both formulate their products almost exclusively from certified organic, raw, whole foods. Herb Pharm is another company that puts quality first, formulating their proprietary herbal compounds from scrupulously selected wild-crafted or certified organic herbs often grown on their own pristine farm in southern Oregon. These companies were founded by visionaries who put human and environmental health before the balance sheet in their business models.

In the much maligned SELECT study, researchers at the Fred Hutchinson Cancer Research Center attempted to determine whether vitamin-E alone or in combination with selenium could prevent prostate cancer. Previous studies had shown 50 IU of natural vitamin E was protective against prostate cancer, but the SELECT study chose to use *synthetic* vitamin E (dl-alpha-tocopherol) at a dosage of 400 IU per day. Results showed that the subjects taking synthetic vitamin E alone had a 17% higher risk of prostate cancer compared to the control group.

After reading the results of the study many questions remain. Renowned family physician and New York Times bestselling author, Dr. Joel Furhman, had more than a few questions for the researchers behind the SELECT study. He published them on Huffington Post: "Were they eating more fish overall? More breaded and fried fish? More large, predator fish? The type of fish and how it is prepared would impact the level of environmental contaminants and dietary carcinogens ... These unanswered questions make it very difficult to extract any useful information from this study's results. For it to have substantive impact they would have had to track dietary fish consumption, fish oil consumption and have confirmed ... blood tests taken episodically." Dr. Furhman asks excellent questions. The answers to which are inexplicably and unforgivably missing from the SELECT report.

Studies with conclusions that run totally opposite to the overwhelming majority of published data need to be carefully scrutinized for methodology and context before they are accepted as true. Suggesting that Omega-3 supplements can cause prostate cancer, when scrutinized carefully, doesn't pass the test of basic common sense. It was a hatchet job, nothing more than misleading junk science. Nonetheless it received widespread media exposure.

If any group was biased and wanted to demonstrate negative results from dietary supplementation, the easiest way would be to study the effects of administering large doses of synthetic vitamins and then make blanket statements that erroneously associate their results with natural supplements.

With Big Pharma controlled healthcare-costs being so high that treating a health crisis is the direct cause of 60% of the personal bankruptcies filed in the US, the old adage, "an once of prevention is worth a pound of cure," has never been more true. For that reason and many others it is my belief that it makes far more sense to address health concerns preemptively, ten years before they've become obvious rather than ten seconds after they've been recognized as a health emergency.

For example, the practice of women including exercise, vitamin D, flaxseed (providing Omega-3 fatty acids), and cruciferous vegetables as part of a healthy lifestyle shows more wisdom than forsaking common sense and then relying on the cancer treatment industry *after* being diagnosed with breast cancer. For men 40 and above, using a natural, synergistic blend of prostate improving nutrients at the very first sign of urinary pattern changes can have immediate and long-term benefits. There is sufficient, good and thorough *real* science to support all of these assertions.

22

Winning The Cold War

"Know The Enemy And Know Yourself" *

Every year, cold and flu viruses must love watching humans preparing for cold and flu season. For viruses, it's a dream come true. It begins in October when we go through the ritual of sealing up our homes for winter – good-bye fresh air, sunshine, and vitamin D – hello stale, recycled air and darkness. Then, we kick off the season with the official American sugar festival supreme - Halloween. Over the next two months our ritualistic over-indulgence of food, alcohol, and sweets carries us through the holiday gauntlet of Thanksgiving and Christmas culminating with the fun of an alcohol saturated, sleep deprived, New Year's celebration - Yee-Haw!!! Add to this the stress of travel, shopping, or being invaded by bands of visiting relatives carrying pathogens from distant lands, and we have done almost everything humanly possible to make ourselves gracious hosts for viruses, patiently waiting to seize fertile opportunities just like this, to celebrate the holiday season in their own special way.

179

In short, relatively affluent folks, who can afford to seriously over-do luxuries, can be their own worst enemy.

In the winter months, everywhere is ground zero and wherever you turn, there's no escape. Anyone who physically interacts with humans is exposed to cold viruses multiple times virtually every day. When exposed, our immune system naturally goes on the offensive and a well rested, properly fed body wins that battle nearly every time, usually without us consciously knowing the fight ever took place.

Experts agree, the basics of a strong immune system are simple: sufficient good quality deep sleep and fueling your body with abundant healthful nutrients are the non-negotiable means to staying healthy. World renowned holistic health practitioners Doctors Michael Murray and Andrew Weil agree that excess sugar and alcohol consumption can severely impair immune response.

When accomplished Western doctors rediscover and embrace ancient Chinese remedies, it's time for the rest of us to pay attention.

Dr. Weil is a Harvard trained MD, has appeared on the cover of Time Magazine twice and was named one of the 100 most influential people in the world. He wrote: "If you tend to get every bug that goes around, you can build up your resistance by using the time-tested Chinese herb Astragalus.* If there was only one herb to take to increase resistance to colds and flus, Astragalus would be it" – it's been the #1 immune enhancing herb used in Traditional Chinese Medicine for centuries and is slightly warming, making it ideal for winter time use.

---

* Please note: because Astragalus is slightly warming, it should not be used if a fever is present.

Doctors at Sloan-Kettering Cancer Institute in New York are also impressed with the immune enhancing qualities of Astragalus. Astragalus is economical, energizing and can be used every day for months at a time.

Nonetheless, the common cold remains the number one reason for work and school absences. So for many, the question inevitably becomes: what to do when a cold virus or its more extreme cousin, a flu virus, starts to win the battle?

Naturally, your body's defenses ramp up and what we consider cold symptoms are actually our immune system fighting the good fight. Harvard Health Publications states: "The miserable symptoms of a cold or the flu are actually signs that your immune system is working to fight off the offending virus. You get a fever, for example, because your immune system's cells work better at a higher body temperature, while germs don't reproduce as well at temperatures above 98.6. The swelling in your sinuses is due to the fact that armies of immune cells are rushing to the area to fight the germs. A runny nose allows your body to flush out germs."

Dr. Fred Pullen, an ear, nose, and throat specialist with over 50 years experience, surprises many with his approach. Patients are referred to Dr. Pullen for the sole purpose of having tubes surgically implanted in their eardrums to help drain pus and backed up fluids. This procedure becomes necessary for some people because their Eustachian tubes clog frequently during colds and ear infections. This prevents drainage and causes painful buildup, a condition more common in children.

Before recommending surgery however, Dr. Pullen places all his patients on a diet that eliminates dairy foods. The result, according to Pullen, is that 75 out of 100 of his patients never need the surgery. A recommendation for a simple, virtually free, method of avoiding surgery, from a doctor who surely makes more \$\$\$ by doing the surgery, demonstrates that Dr. Pullen is a healer with high integrity.

The foundation of staying healthy and preventing colds and flus is built on the daily basics such as: taking a high quality, whole-food multivitamin and extra vitamin D, along with getting moderate physical activity, fresh air, pure water and most importantly, sufficient, deep sleep. The importance of avoiding excess alcohol, sugar and other dietary extremes is also undeniable. Notice that everything listed are factors many people conveniently disregard in the holiday season but are nonetheless within our power to easily influence to our advantage.

One important fact to remember is that antibiotics have absolutely no effect on viruses. Despite this fact, 60% of doctors prescribe antibiotics to their patients suffering from severe cold and flu viruses. The following suggestions offer natural perspectives on battling colds and flu.

Chinese Medicine generally views colds as surface, therefore less serious, illnesses. The theory is that from the surface it can more easily travel outward. The goal is to cure it quickly before it travels to deeper regions of the body. An ancient Chinese herbal formula called Yin Chiao (pronounced chow) was created to do that. The diaphoretic herbs in Yin Chiao help warm the body's surface, induce sweating, and help bring pathogens up and out. Using Yin Chaio, I usually feel a little warm and slightly uncomfortable for a few hours and then my cold symptoms typically disappear.

There have been over 300 scientific investigations of the immune-enhancing effects of Echinacea. Using sufficient quantities of a high quality extract, prepared from freshly harvested E. purpurea echinacea plants produced excellent results. Dosing 10 times the first day and four times the following days has been shown to reduce symptoms, severity, and duration significantly compared to the placebo. Lower doses or using products made from old or dried leaves proved substantially less effective.

Folklore surrounding elderberry for treating flu is legendary. In addition, scientists in Israel showed that elderberry created dramatic improvements in virtually all flu symptoms. After the first day of use, 20% of those receiving elderberry felt relief. By day three, 90% of the treated group showed improvements compared to only 16% of the untreated group who took nearly a week to improve. Dr. Russell Greenfield, MD, director of Carolinas Integrative Health, concurs and wrote in a news release, "Black Elderberry is effective and can be given to children and adults, and with no known side effects or negative interactions."

More than a dozen placebo-controlled clinical trials have examined the therapeutic effect of zinc lozenges on the common cold. The results demonstrate up to a 42% reduction in the duration of colds using daily doses of 75 milligrams. On average, complete recovery was achieved in 4.4 days versus 7.6 days for the placebo. Dissolving zinc gluconate in water, gargling, swallowing, and following up with zinc lozenges throughout the day is good way to receive your 75mg. If lozenges are used, for maximum effectiveness, they should be free of citric acid and the sweeteners manitol and sorbitol.

Traditional Medicinals Tea Company has formulated some highly effective herbal blends for treating cold symptoms. **Herbatussin Cough Tea, Throat Coat, Cold Care PM and Breathe Easy** are four of the most effective formulas available. They come in convenient, pre-blended tea bags and are **extremely** economical. They're available in many health food and some grocery stores.

Stocking your natural medicine (war) chest with these items is a great way to gain the strategic advantage in this year's cold and flu battles.

*Sun Tzu, author of <u>The Art of War</u>, was a Chinese military general, strategist, and philosopher who lived around 500 BC. One of his book's most enduring quotes is: "If you know the enemy and know yourself, you need not fear the result of a hundred battles." Knowing that cold and flu viruses often thrive in human bodies that have been made overly acidic by poor diet, lack of proper rest and fresh air, and/or excess, stress and alcohol, should give you the decided advantage when preparing for cold and flu season. Simply change the battleground conditions and gain the advantage.

23

Natural Birthing And Baby Care

My Kids Were Born At A Crime Scene

Natural childbirth is empowering for mothers and reaffirms that they are the ultimate authority about their child's health and well-being. Yet in the 1980s, when our kids were born in Massachusetts, the medical lobbies were successful in making midwifery assisted home-births illegal. Nonetheless, my wife chose to deliver our four children at home with a midwife's help. **Legally, I guess that means our kids were born at a crime scene**. Thankfully the statute of limitations on our "criminal activity" has run out and we can speak freely without fear of legal consequences.

Let's Examine This Subject In Three Parts:

1) Birthing Has Become Big Business
2) Who's Feeding the Kids?
3) Natural Baby Formula Recipe For Those Times A Supplement To Breast Milk Is Needed

Part 1) Birthing Has Become Big Business

Today, less than one percent of all births nationwide take place at home, and midwifery is still illegal in 11 states. Elise Hanson, a certified midwife practicing in Eugene, Oregon stated the problem: "There's a lot of friction between the medical model and the midwifery model. Our system doesn't allow a working relationship between midwives and doctors." She cites the Netherlands as a case study in effective, integrative birthing practices. Thirty-five percent of babies are born at home in the Netherlands, and the relationship between midwives and doctors is cooperative, not competitive.

The Huffington Post reported: "The United States spends $98 billion annually on hospitalization for pregnancy and childbirth, **but the US maternal mortality rate has doubled in the past 25 years.** The US medical system ranks 50th in the world for maternal mortality, meaning that the medical systems in 49 countries were better at keeping late stage pregnant women and new mothers alive."

About one third of babies born in the US are now delivered by C-section (Cesarean). Dr. George A. Macones, a spokesman for the American College of Obstetricians and Gynecologists said: **"The increased tendency to induce labor with drugs before a woman's due date, for reasons of convenience, has helped push up the Cesarean rate, because inducing labor with drugs is more likely, than natural labor, to fail and result in a Cesarean.** We should do chemical inductions for good solid medical reasons, not for convenience or the day of the week." Elective C-sections keep doctors from having to deliver babies

186

nights, weekends, holidays, or other times that may be inconvenient for **them**.

Maternal deaths were a much more common tragedy 100 years ago but after nearly a century of reductions in serious birthing complications, rates have risen sharply. In 1987, there were 6.6 maternal deaths per 100,000 births in the US; today there are 16.7. Necessary Cesareans can certainly save lives, but no matter how common this procedure gets, it's still major surgery. And with that comes major risks - pulmonary embolism, infection, hemorrhage, etc., and it can increase placental complications in future pregnancies. So the risk doesn't end with the current pregnancy. **Countries that have the highest C-section rates also have the highest maternal death rates.** I don't think that's a coincidence. Technology can be lifesaving, but overuse of that technology can be counterproductive.

Some states are getting it right. In Massachusetts a majority of the state's birth centers recently banned elective C-sections and chemically induced labor except when there is a clear medical need. The move was based on numerous studies that found that such policies led to reductions in stillbirths and serious birth-related complications.

Another aim of the hospitals' new rules is to shorten the time a pregnant woman spends laboring in the hospital, which frees up beds and saves on healthcare costs. Women who go into labor naturally tend to spend about 10.5 hours in the labor and delivery unit compared with 22 hours for women whose labor is induced with drugs.

Allowing nature to take its course is safer and ultimately more economical.

Average total cost of giving birth in different ways:

- Midwife assisted at home or at a birthing center $2,000 to $3,000
- Hospital vaginal birth $9,000
- C-section, over $20,000

The Centers for Disease Control recently reported that home births have increased 20% in the past four years. Studies cite the steady increase of Cesarean sections, and their high cost, as reasons women are avoiding hospital births.

The mere fact that the Centers for *DISEASE* Control is in charge of monitoring data for this natural process says a lot about medical attitudes in the US surrounding birth.

Part 2) Who's Feeding the Babies?

During the past 100 years, infant nutrition, child care, and family structure have undergone the most profound changes in human history, with much of that occurring right here in the United States. In 1900, six percent of married women worked outside the home, usually only when their blue-collar husbands were unemployed. Among women with young children, few ever worked away from home. Since then, the percentage of women who work outside the home has increased tenfold.

With so many women now in the workforce, who's feeding the kids? Back in the fifties, misguided doctors regularly recommended feeding infants laboratory prepared, store bought formulas because it was thought to be more "hygienic and scientific." Fortunately, the American Academy of Pediatrics now recommends breastfeeding for the first 12 months of life. The lifelong benefits transferred to the baby are so numerous, that this subject deserves its own exclusive book. For moms holding down jobs outside the home, breastfeeding is not always easy but it remains the most appropriate way to nourish young humans.

In America, bringing kids to work and breastfeeding there, is nearly unheard of. Some women pump and refrigerate or freeze their own breast milk so childcare providers can later feed it to their baby. But that process is cumbersome, and sometimes leaving the baby for a full work shift causes milk production to diminish. If this happens, other food is needed – that becomes tricky.

Feeding human infants milk from other animals is far from an ideal solution. Bovine calves grow 500% to 600% in year one, so cow's milk is relatively high in protein and calcium to support that physical growth. Mother seals make a high-fat milk because baby seals need lots of body fat to survive in cold water. Human babies have different needs. Their physical size increases only two to three times, but their intelligence gains in their first year are astronomical. Consequently, human milk is appropriately lower in protein but far richer in fats, sugars and other nutrients that support brain development and function. This principle is known as the biological specificity of milk.

Though the protein content of human milk is generally low, the types of amino acids that make up these proteins are important. One particular amino acid, taurine, is found in large amounts in human milk. Studies show that taurine has an important role for humans in the development of the brain and the eyes. The body cannot convert other kinds of amino acids into taurine, so its presence in human milk is significant.

Adult foods can be ground or blended to be swallowed by toothless babies, but their digestive tracts lack many of the enzymes needed to digest and assimilate adult foods. Store bought infant formulas designed to replace breast milk fall short in many areas, some easily measured and some not. They often contain ingredients that are difficult for some babies to digest. Parents who have ever fed their formula to their baby and then listened to them cry all night with a bellyache know this well.

Dr. William Sears, parenting and child nutrition guru, writing about high fructose corn syrup (HFCS) in formulas stated: "that ingredient is not used because of any health benefits, but because it is sweeter and cheaper to produce." Dr. Sears further states: "the number one cause of the childhood obesity epidemic is the over consumption of HFCS, mainly in the form of beverages."

Nothing remotely approaches the perfection, on every level, of a healthy mother breastfeeding her baby. Mother's milk even changes over time as the baby's needs change. For example, the first milk a mother supplies to its baby in the first hours and days of life is colostrum. The concentration of immune factors is much higher in colostrum than in milk produced in the ensuing months. This helps keep the baby healthy by programming the newborn's immune system.

Mother's milk is virtually always the best option. But when it's necessary to use supplemental nutrition, here is a healthy, natural recipe for homemade infant formula I created for our family and have seen used with great success by others as well.

Top considerations for this formula were organic ingredients, correct nutrient balance for human babies and digestibility. Babies really like it and digest it well with no gas, colic, crying, or unusually smelly diapers.

Part 3) Natural Baby Formula Recipe, For Those Times A Supplement To Breast Milk Is Needed

- ⅄ 1 cup each, organic: long grain brown rice, short grain brown rice, sweet brown rice, oat groats, quinoa
- ⅄ Three or Four, 4-inch pieces of dried Kombu seaweed
- ⅄ Soak grains in pure water for 4-8 hours. In a total of about 15 cups of water, using an, 8-quart stainless steel pressure cooker, cook the grains with the Kombu for 45 minutes. (exercise caution when using pressure cookers).
- ⅄ After the pressure comes completely down, remove lid and add:
- ⅄ 1 1/2 Tablespoons each:
- ⅄ Organic extra virgin coconut oil
- ⅄ Organic highest lignan flax oil (pure fish oil might substitute here but I've never tried it)
- ⅄ Let mixture cool 1-2 hours
- ⅄ Empty and stir into the mixture the contents of one capsule of a premium, high potency full spectrum, digestive enzyme (or 2-3 low potency capsules)
- ⅄ Let sit about 30 minutes
- ⅄ Grind it with a hand crank food mill. Electric blenders infuse the mix with air which can create digestive challenges. Strain the mixture twice.
- ⅄ Use immediately, refrigerate or freeze for future use. Best served at baby temperature, 98.6 degrees.

This formula is an excellent *adjunct* to mother's milk and that is the only way I have seen it used for extended periods. Please note that it probably contains insufficient protein to be used as a stand-alone formula for prolonged use. For extended use as the majority of the baby's diet, it would be wise to to add protein powder to the mix as well – a raw, plant-based, soy-free blend or whey protein are my recommendations. Try them out in different batches and see which one you think is best for your baby.

Raw goat's milk may be another viable option.

The processes surrounding natural child birth and baby feeding had been used successfully on approximately 80 to 90 billion test subjects before the modern medical system decided we needed a "new-normal." Are we really sure that expensive and often invasive interventions are better for mother and baby? We should have the complete results of this modern experiment in a thousand years or so. In the meantime, I'll continue to recommend Mother Nature as the most qualified expert in this field of study.

24

Vaccines: What Your Doctor Won't Tell You

Extensive Misinformation Abounds

The vaccine rate has skyrocketed in the last 30 years. Virtually any medical doctor is more than happy to provide a long list of reasons they think children should be vaccinated. **Current American Academy of Pediatrics recommendations state that children should receive 35 vaccine doses by the age of 15 months, 49 doses by the age of six, and 69 doses by the age of 18.** Although they are usually represented as mandatory, it is important to note that vaccination is an elective procedure.

Included in those recommendations, is that parents begin vaccinating their children the day they're born for Hepatitis B, a disease that is transmitted sexually or through shared needle use. Why? **Because the misinformation surrounding vaccination is so extensive, many parents don't even question whether or not they should vaccinate their child. However, parents should view these as very major decisions.** The lifelong health and well-being of their child may depend

193

on the critical decisions parents make in this area.

A logical look at disease and vaccine statistics may surprise many. Unfortunately, most people are not exposed to all the facts before they're convinced to accept vaccine injections. In every mature decision we make in life we need to consider two things: The potential upside gain, if all goes well, versus, the possible down-side risk.

From the Centers for Disease Control (CDC) website. The number of vaccine doses recommended by the age of 15 months:

DPT (3 vaccines in one) 4 times	= 12
HiB 4 times	= 4
Pneumococcal 4 times	= 4
Hep B 3 times	= 3
polio 3 times	= 3
rotavirus 3 times	= 3
MMR (3 vaccines in one) 1 time	= 3
influenza 2 times	= 2
varicella (chicken pox) 1 time	= 1
Total	**= 35**

To be as logical and clear as possible, let's study this important subject in five basic parts:

1) **Historical Vaccine Data**

2) **Effectiveness: Have vaccines been proven to work?**

3) **Safety: What are the likely or potential unwanted side-effects?**

4) **Natural ways to safely enhance immunity, with or without vaccines**

5) **Conclusion**

Part 1: Historical Vaccine Data

The term vaccine comes from *vacca*, the Latin word for cow. In 1796 the first modern vaccine was created when diseased infectious material from cow pox, a disease affecting cows' udders, was injected into humans to protect them from contracting smallpox, a related disease that occurs in humans. Unfortunately, deaths from smallpox rose dramatically about 20 years after the vaccine became compulsory.

Many people might be surprised to learn that the incidence of virtually all infectious diseases declined significantly *before* the introduction of vaccines. In the US and England, the death rate from Pertussis (whooping cough) dropped from about 60 deaths per thousand in the mid 1800s to about two per thousand in the early 1950s, even before the Pertussis vaccine was used. Deaths from measles from the mid 1800s until the 1963 introduction of the measles vaccine fell at a nearly identical rate.

In both cases, even before the introduction of the vaccines, the death rate from these diseases had already fallen approximately 97% - this according to data extracted from public health records and published by Roman Bystrianyk and Suzanne Humphries MD in their exceptional book, <u>Dissolving Illusions: Disease, Vaccines, and the Forgotten History</u>.

According to international mortality statistics, from about 1925 until 1955, the 30 years *before* the first polio vaccine was invented, the polio death rate had already dropped about 50% in the US and England. However, in the year immediately following the introduction of the polio vaccine, the death rate from polio rose significantly.

Government statistics reported by the Associated Press in 1955, the year after the polio vaccine was invented and widely administered, stated the death rate from polio *increased*, on average, 530% in the states of Vermont, New Hampshire, Massachusetts, Connecticut and Rhode Island. Fortunately the rate later continued on the documented downward trend that began decades before the vaccine was introduced.

Polio has since essentially disappeared in the US and throughout Europe, even in the European countries that had no mass vaccination programs. Internationally respected pediatrician, Dr. Robert Mendelsohn stated that, "the disease simply ran its course."

The 1850s appears to be the turning point when death rates from many infectious diseases began to drop sharply. I think this is directly related to two important milestones. Based on groundbreaking research from Hungarian physician, Dr. Ignaz Semmelweis, and later confirmed by Luis Pasteur and Joseph Lister, doctors became aware of the life saving benefits of washing their hands between patients. Then around 1900, municipalities began disinfecting drinking water. **When these two aspects of basic modern hygiene became the norm, data irrefutably demonstrates death rates from infectious diseases plummeted,** *long* **before most vaccines were introduced.**

Research from 1913 Nobel Prize winner in medicine, Dr. Charles Richet, demonstrated that hay fever, asthma, anaphylactic shock and other inflammatory allergic reactions were often caused by reactions to undigested proteins introduced into the bloodstream by injected vaccines. Ask your doctor if she has even heard of this groundbreaking 100-year-old research. Then ask why medical schools don't teach about Richet's work. The answer: Big Pharma doesn't want it taught.

Some researchers now believe that trace proteins from peanut oil, a common ingredient in many vaccines, is the likely cause of otherwise unexplained deadly peanut allergies. **This explains why children who have never before eaten peanuts can experience deadly reactions the first time they eat the food.** It's probably because their immune systems were already in hyper-drive reacting to undigested peanut proteins that had bypassed the digestive tract - being injected directly into the bloodstream. It's also totally consistent with Richet's discoveries.

Like Richet's Nobel Prize winning research, unbiased studies from qualified researchers are desperately needed so the general public and medical communities can get accurate data on which to base informed vaccine decisions.

Part 2: Vaccine Effectiveness: Do They Work?

Vaccines are supposed to fool your body's immune system into believing it is facing a real threat from a viral or bacterial infection. It is thought that the antibodies your body was tricked into producing will help it become immune to future infection from the disease.

Because vaccines are used predominately on children, most people assume that all vaccines have been subjected to thorough, rigorous testing and trials proving that they are effective and safe. However, parents have wrongly been told, as discussed in the history portion above, that mass vaccination campaigns ended multiple epidemics around the world.

Taking the time to logically review pro-vaccine assertions, we find that they lack solid scientific backing. Not only has there never been a single long-term scientific study comparing the health and welfare of vaccinated to unvaccinated children, multiple examples can easily be found of vaccinated children acquiring the very illness they have been vaccinated against.

Even if parents find out about the risks of vaccines on their own, their doctors usually assure them that the risk is worth the almost certain, alleged benefit of freedom from infectious disease that their child supposedly receives. However, time and again, the facts are that vaccines have simply not worked against the diseases they are targeted to prevent.

The medical literature is filled with example after example of the failure of vaccination to furnish protection against common childhood diseases.

Mumps used to be a routine childhood illness. Typically the virus ran its course while you stayed at home in bed, and in return, you received lifelong immunity. In virtually all cases of mumps, like many of the childhood illnesses we're now vaccinating children against, it is not a serious disease.

In the United States, children typically receive their mumps vaccination as part of the Measles, Mumps, and Rubella (MMR) vaccine. The US Centers for Disease Control and Prevention (CDC) advises that children receive their first dose between 12 and 18 months, and their second between the ages of 4 and 6 years.

In late 2009, over 1,000 people in NJ were sickened with the mumps. Public health officials there linked the outbreak to an 11-year old boy who had been fully vaccinated against the disease <u>as had 77% of those who became ill.</u>

This MMR vaccine is supposed to make people immune to measles, mumps and rubella… yet in 2009, 77% of the 1,000+ who were sickened with mumps in one community were vaccinated.

A 1990 *Journal of American Medicine Association* (JAMA) article stated that, "Although more than 95% of school-aged children in the US are vaccinated against measles, large measles outbreaks continue to occur in schools and most cases occur among previously vaccinated children." A 1978 survey of 30 states showed that more than half of all children who contracted measles had been fully vaccinated.

In 1984, the CDC confirmed that a measles outbreak occurred in an Illinois high school where 100% of students had been vaccinated.

In 1985, the *New England Journal of Medicine* reported that an outbreak of measles occurred among adolescents in Corpus Christi, Texas, even though more than 99% had records of vaccination with live measles vaccine.

In 1988, an outbreak of 84 measles cases occurred at a college in Colorado in which over 98% of students had documentation of what was thought to be adequate measles immunity according to a report published in the *American Journal of Public Health*.

Even though the MMR vaccine offers questionable protection for three diseases that were never particularly dangerous, there can still be an incredibly steep price to pay for receiving it. As of March 1, 2012, there had been 898 claims filed in the federal Vaccine Injury Compensation Program (VICP) for serious injuries and deaths following MMR vaccination.

The DPT triple vaccine (diphtheria, pertussis, and tetanus) is supposed to convey immunity to pertussis (whooping cough). In 2010, the largest outbreak of whooping cough in over 50 years reportedly occurred in California. What appears to have been a scare campaign was then launched in the state by Big Pharma funded medical trade associations and public health officials, falsely accusing people who had opted-out of the pertussis vaccine as being the cause of that whooping cough outbreak.

But research released in 2012 painted a very different picture than what had been spread by the media in 2010.

In a study published in *Clinical Infectious Diseases*, researchers reviewed data on every patient under 18 years old who tested positive for pertussis between March and October 2010 at the Kaiser Permanente Medical Center in San Rafael, California. Out of these 132 patients:

- ⅄ **81 percent were fully up to date on the whooping cough vaccine**
- ⅄ **8 percent had never been vaccinated**
- ⅄ **11 percent had received at least one shot, but not the entire recommended series**

In 1994, the *New England Journal of Medicine* reported that during a pertussis outbreak in Ohio, 82% of younger children stricken with the disease had received regular doses of the vaccine.

In 1978, studies in Sweden examined 5,140 cases of whooping cough (pertussis) in that country and found that 84% of those afflicted had received at least three rounds of the pertussis vaccine.

Before the day that your family's pediatrician asks your child to roll up his/her sleeve, ask for reasonable explanations for the failures discussed above. What data will they offer that *scientifically* demonstrates vaccine effectiveness? Whatever they offer, take it home and study it carefully before making your decision.

Many laypeople and physicians look to the National Centers for Disease Control (CDC) in Atlanta for definitive answers about health issues including answers to questions about vaccines. Below is a verbatim answer from the CDC website to the straightforward question:

How Effective Is The Flu Vaccine? This Answer Is Directly From The CDC Website:

"At least two factors play an important role in determining the likelihood that flu vaccine will protect a person from flu illness: 1) characteristics of the person being vaccinated (such as their age and health), and 2) the similarity or "match" between the flu viruses the flu vaccine is designed to protect against and the flu viruses spreading in the community. During years when the flu vaccine is not well matched to circulating viruses, it's possible that no benefit from flu vaccination may be observed. During years when there is a good match between the flu vaccine and circulating viruses, it's possible to measure substantial benefits from vaccination in terms of preventing flu illness. However, even during years when the vaccine match is very good, the benefits of vaccination will vary across the

population, depending on characteristics of the person being vaccinated and even, potentially, which vaccine was used."

To sum up their answers: There is no way for a doctor or layperson to know if the flu shot being administered matches up with the flus that are actual threats in any given year. The years when it doesn't match up, it's ***possible*** that there will be no benefit whatsoever (I personally believe that possibility is actually a virtual 100% certainty).

The CDC claims that during years when the vaccine matches up with the actual flu threat, "it's *possible* to measure substantial benefit." **Notice they don't say benefit *has* been measured.** The only way benefit could be scientifically measured is with a placebo-controlled double blind study, i.e. administer the vaccine to some, while administering a placebo to a statistically similar control group. The CDC website states that studies of this type are ***not*** done because it would be unethical to deprive some people of the possible benefits of flu vaccine. Further, they don't define the words *substantial benefit.* Would a *substantial benefit* be a 2%, 5%, or 15% reduction in flu cases? They don't say, so the intelligent among us are left guessing what they might be implying.

The CDC website further states: *"In general, the flu vaccine works best among healthy adults and children older than 2 years of age. Reduced benefits of flu vaccine are often found in studies of young children (e.g., those younger than 2 years of age) and older adults (e.g., adults 65 years of age and older)."*

They have to say *in general,* because they have no definitive studies. But it's ironic that, ***if*** there is any benefit at all, people most at risk from serious flu complications, the elderly and the

202

very young, are the ones who can expect the least benefit. And *if* there is any benefit at all, it could only possibly occur during years when the vaccine and the flu are a match. But, since for so-called ethical reasons, they won't do any truly scientific testing; we'll never know *if* any of their theories on flu vaccines have any validity whatsoever, despite an annual price tag of approximately two billion dollars.

From another so-called authoritative source, The National Network For Immunization Information, the answer to the simple question:

Because Of Better Hygiene and Sanitation, Hadn't Diseases Already Begun To Disappear Before Vaccines Were Introduced?

Answer directly from their website:

"No, they had not begun to disappear. In the 20th century, infectious diseases began to be better controlled because of improvements in hygiene and sanitation (clean water and pest control). However, the incidence of vaccine-preventable diseases only began to drop dramatically after the vaccines for those diseases were licensed and began to be used in large numbers of children."

Their answer directly contradicts all official public health data available which clearly demonstrates that many diseases that vaccines were created to eliminate had already been reduced by 97% before the vaccines were even invented. This is conclusively documented in the brilliant book by Bystrianyk and Humphries mentioned above.

The assertions made by the National Network For Immunization Information don't pass a basic sniff test and are equal parts asinine and sad, and if we traced their funding sources, possibly unethical.

The medical experts have confusing, convoluted answers inconsistent with accepted historical data. They refuse to do scientific testing. But rather than even *consider* **the possibility that the system of vaccination could be seriously flawed, the medical industry simply calls for "booster" shots and re-vaccination, without any solid, long-term studies to see whether immunity is actually achieved and, if so, for how long.**

Whereas natural recovery from many infectious diseases stimulates lifetime immunity from one bout with the disease, vaccines only provide (at best) temporary protection, proven by the fact that most vaccines now require "booster" doses to extend the alleged, vaccine-induced, man-made immunity.

So if you are trying to do your own risk/reward analysis about whether or not to vaccinate, how can you be really sure what the reward is? The CDC certainly isn't and they claim it would be unethical to do scientific studies to find out.

Part 3: Vaccine Safety

Most doctors are happy to administer whatever vaccines producers claim are safe but are reluctant to discuss the fact that the for-profit vaccine manufacturers are legally protected from lawsuit should their products prove to be harmful or deadly. They can pump out anything they want with no financial risk at all. **I can think of no other for-profit business that**

is absolved of all legal liability for the safety or effectiveness of their products.

Vaccines typically introduce lab-altered live viruses and killed bacteria into the human body along with chemicals, metals, drugs, and other additives such as formaldehyde, aluminum, mercury, monosodium glutamate, sodium phosphate, phenoxyethanol, gelatin, sulfites, peanut protein, yeast protein, antibiotics as well as unknown amounts of RNA and DNA from animal and human cell tissue cultures. And IF a parent follows current American Academy of Pediatrics recommendations, they will be allowing a doctor to inject 49 doses of these mystery combinations into their child by age six.

Mainstream medical professionals offer no proven explanations of why autism rates have risen to 1 in 50 except to say those outrageously high numbers can easily be explained away solely by differences in reporting methodology. Additionally, serious ADHD issues, acute allergies, asthma, cancer, and autoimmune disease rates have all substantially increased in kids in the past 30 years, according to Centers For Disease Control and The American Lung Association. **In 1994, the *Journal of the American Medical Association* published data showing that children diagnosed with asthma were five times more likely than not to have received the pertussis vaccine.** While they can track the growth of these maladies, medical professionals offer no reasonable explanation for the increase. We definitely need unbiased scientific studies. Instead we get assumptions.

The time honored (common sense based) rule that pregnant women should avoid unnecessary exposure to potential toxins such as alcohol, cigarette smoke, medications, radiation, household cleaning products, etc. was inexplicably replaced in 2006 by an *assumption* that the toxins present in vaccines are completely safe for developing fetuses. That is when the Centers for Disease Control (CDC) strengthened recommendations that *all* pregnant women, healthy or not, should get a flu shot in *any* trimester. Then, in 2011, a pertussis containing shot (Tdap: tetanus, diptheria, pertussis) was recommended for *all* pregnant women. Both current vaccine recommendations are endorsed by the American Congress of Obstetricians and Gynecologists and the American Academy of Pediatrics, without any safety studies to back these arbitrary recommendations.

Fact: The Food and Drug Administration (FDA) lists influenza and Tdap vaccines as either Pregnancy Category B or C biologicals, which means that *adequate testing has <u>not</u> been done* in humans to demonstrate safety for pregnant women and it is not known whether the vaccines can cause fetal harm or affect reproduction capacity. *Even the manufacturers* of influenza and Tdap vaccines state that human toxicity and fertility studies are inadequate and warn that the influenza and Tdap vaccines should "be given to a pregnant woman only if clearly needed."

The CDC, *shoot-first-ask-questions-later,* policy is another obvious example ill-conceived, profit-first vaccine policy placing science and the health of humans in second place

In 2011, a study was published in the peer reviewed journal, *Human & Experimental Toxicology*, exposing the alarming relationship between vaccinating and infant mortality. Of the 34 countries studied, **the United States ranked 34th (worst) in infant mortality and topped the list for the most vaccines administered under one year of age.** The countries of the world that vaccinated least had the lowest infant mortality and the countries that vaccinated the most had higher rates.

Many adverse events are not reported or tracked. One of the great dangers of the current pro-vaccine mentality is the fact that negative vaccine reactions are very rarely reported to the adverse event reporting system - a system rife with problems. When a vaccine is released onto the market, post-marketing surveillance is supposed to track any negative reactions from the millions of people taking the newly released vaccine. However, not only is the adverse reporting system entirely voluntary, 90 to 99 percent of all adverse reactions are never reported, according to David Kessler, former head of the FDA under presidents George H.W. Bush and Bill Clinton. With regards to any reports that are made directly to the pharmaceutical companies, there is absolutely no accountability mechanism to ensure that that data is ever forwarded to the FDA - **the process is run entirely by the *"honor system."***

To aid vaccine makers, in the mid-1980s, Congress removed legal liability from them for damage done by unwanted vaccine side-effects. This occurred after the manufacturers testified the financial impact from injury awards, stemming primarily from bad reactions to the DPT triple vaccine (diphtheria, pertussis and tetanus), had threatened their existence. However, because the possibility of severe harm or death resulting from vaccines was so obvious, in 1988 Congress set up an alternate system for vaccine victims to receive compensation – the National Vaccine Injury Compensation Program, (NVICP), commonly known as *The Vaccine Court.* But it is not actually a court, it's a federal no-fault compensation system utilizing "special masters" employed by the Federal Government instead of judges. **To date the Vaccine**

Court has awarded nearly three billion dollars to victims of serious vaccine side effects. In the last four years awards have averaged over $225,000,000 annually and so far in 2014 awards are on a record pace that, if continued, will be nearly double that. However, it's a no-fault system. So when evidence proves someone was damaged from a tainted or problematic vaccine, or even one that performed as designed, the vaccine makers pay nothing and receive no sanctions. It's ironic to note that the vast majority of vaccine injury awards in the Vaccine Court have, so far, been for children suffering DPT vaccine induced brain injuries and deaths.

There is a huge volume of evidence proving that side effects from vaccines are far more serious and common than the vaccine manufacturers willingly admit. Since the manufacturers downplay the truth, there is almost no way for most doctors to find accurate data. It's well documented that Big Pharma provides high dollar grants, typically in the tens of millions per year, per school, for most of the major medical schools in the US. Doctors are indoctrinated during their years in school with no way of knowing who is controlling the facts they are coerced into memorizing.

As Barbara Loe Fisher, president and co-founder of the National Vaccine Information Center, states: *"The fact that man-made vaccines cannot replicate the body's natural experience with the disease is one of the key points of contention between those who insist that mankind cannot live without mass use of multiple vaccines and those who believe that mankind's biological integrity will be severely compromised by their continued use."*

Loe Fisher further explains it comes down to weighing the possible upside benefit:

"First, is it better to (possibly) *protect children against infectious disease early in life through temporary immunity from a vaccine or are they better off contracting certain contagious infections in childhood and attaining permanent immunity?"*

Versus the downside risk:

"Second, do vaccine complications ultimately cause more chronic illness and death than infectious diseases do? Both questions essentially pit trust in human intervention against trust in nature and the natural order, which existed long before vaccines were created by man."

Some researchers have begun to attribute the huge increase in autism to air pollution and other environmental factors, often deflecting discussion away from vaccines. I believe that it's likely that bad food, bad air and other factors are, more than anything else, exacerbating the damage already done by vaccines. These environmental factors are likely to have a much more severe effect on a person whose immune system has already been hyper-sensitized by being exposed to the concentrated toxins in vaccines.

Over millions of years, through adaptation and/or evolution, the human body has developed a supremely efficient and thorough immune system. It is seldom defeated. The primary way to naturally access the human bloodstream is through the digestive track. What you put in your mouth eventually gets absorbed through the intestinal lining and into the bloodstream.

By forcibly injecting vaccines acknowledged to contain toxic substances *directly* into your bloodstream, your doctor completely circumvents four critical ways the immune system avoids and removes inappropriate or potentially toxic substances before they can enter the bloodstream. Injections do the following:

- Bypass the brain's decision-making ability to decide if something looks, feels, smells and tastes good enough to allow it through the gate (mouth), into the system
- Bypass the gag reflex, if your body is grossed out by toxic stuff and wants to spit it out before swallowing
- Bypass the stomach and its ability to throw the whole mess back up in a last ditch effort to protect the intestines from exposure
- And finally, bypass the intestine's ability to avoid toxins by quickly passing it as diarrhea

The skin is the largest part of the body's immune system. Bypassing it with a hypodermic needle your family doctor is essentially declaring that in his 4 years of medical school he has learned enough to confidently override mother nature's finely honed wisdom – not once, but 49 times by the time his patient (your child) is six years old!

Willfully forcing toxic materials that would not likely make it past the normal gatekeepers is a formula to create a hypersensitive immune system that can react, sometimes violently and way out of proportion to the actual threat. This is consistent with the 1913, Nobel Prize Winning conclusions of Dr. Charles Richet (stated earlier in this chapter). Another name for irrational immune system overreaction is, autoimmune disease – like asthma, acute allergies, and many cancers – the very issues that have increased dramatically in children in the last 30 years as the rates of vaccinations have exploded.

> To more thoroughly understand vaccine consequences and effectiveness I strongly recommend the resources offered at the end of this chapter.

Part 4: Natural Ways To Safely Enhance Immunity, With Or Without Vaccines

Western medicine operates under the assumption that synthetic, genetically engineered drugs and vaccines heal the sick and protect the young from disease, an assumption that parents are expected to accept without question. But when it comes to your child, you are the expert most qualified to decide what is best for your child, using your intelligence and common sense in the same way we fight for our right for real food.

When it comes to taking personal responsibility for our health, we should understand many important factors that doctors seldom publicize:

Abundant beneficial bacteria in the gut are a major part of the human immune system and essential for optimum health. Often, after completing a round of antibiotics many people become much more susceptible to reinfection and getting sick from other bacteria and viruses. This occurs because the antibiotics indiscriminately kill all bacteria, good and bad, thereby disrupting an important part of our natural defenses. Digestion and immunity problems after using antibiotics can usually be averted by ingesting premium probiotics to re-seed the gut with essential bacteria following antibiotic use. Probiotics can be found in naturally fermented traditional foods like miso, yogurt, sauerkraut, kim chee, and kefir, as well as in store-bought capsules and liquids. Learn more about probiotics in chapter 25.

The importance of breast milk in protecting the newborn from infection is now recognized worldwide. It's the single best thing any mother can do to enhance her baby's immune system. Specific and nonspecific factors are transferred to the newborn through breast milk and colostrum. The most important role for breast milk in the baby's defense against infection appears to be the supply of local protective factors to the gut through the support of intestinal flora.

In the US, back in the 1950s, many misguided doctors regularly recommended feeding infants laboratory prepared, store bought formulas because it was thought to be more "hygienic and scientific" than breastfeeding. However, lab created imitation formulas do nothing to enhance immune system strength. Fortunately, the American Academy of Pediatrics now recommends breastfeeding for the first 12 months of life.

Avoiding injections should be considered. In 1995, the *New England Journal of Medicine* published a study showing that children who received a single vaccine injection within one month after receiving a polio vaccine were eight times more likely to contract polio than children who received no injections. The risk jumped 27-fold when children received up to nine injections within one month after receiving the polio vaccine. And with ten or more injections, the likelihood of developing polio was 182 times greater than expected. Why injections increase the risk of polio is unclear. Nevertheless, studies indicate that "injections must be avoided in countries with widespread polio."

Nutritional imbalances should not be ignored. A poor diet has also been shown to increase susceptibility to many diseases, including polio. The following excerpt is from Neil Miller's book, Vaccines, Are they Really Safe & Effective?

Does Sugar Consumption Weaken The Immune System?

In 1948, during the height of the polio epidemics, Dr. Benjamin Sandler, a nutritional expert at the Oteen Veterans' Hospital in Asheville, North Carolina, documented a relationship between polio and an excessive use of sugars and starches. He compiled records showing that countries with the highest per capita consumption of sugar, such as the United States, Britain, Australia, Canada, and Sweden (with over 100 pounds per person per year) had the greatest incidence of polio. In contrast, polio was practically unheard of in China (with its sugar use of only 3 pounds per person per year).

Dr. Sandler observed that children consume greater amounts of ice cream, soft drinks, and sugar sweetened products in hot weather. In 1949, before the polio season began, he warned the residents of North Carolina, through the newspapers and radio, to decrease their consumption of these products. That summer, North Carolinians reduced their intake of sugar by 90 percent and polio decreased by the same amount. The North Carolina State Health Department reported 2,498 cases of polio in 1948, and 229 cases in 1949 (data taken from North Carolina State Health Department figures).

One manufacturer shipped one million less gallons of ice cream during the first week alone following the publication of Dr. Sandler's anti-polio diet. Soft drink sales were down as well. But the powerful Rockefeller Milk Trust, which sold frozen products to North Carolinians, combined forces with soft drink business leaders and ran a PR campaign to convince the people that Sandler's findings were a myth and the polio figures a fluke. By the summer of 1950 sales of high sugar products were back to previous levels and polio cases returned to "normal."

– Neil Miller. <u>Vaccines, Are They Really Safe and Effective?</u>

Does the history above prove that Dr. Sandler's theory about the link between sugar consumption and susceptibility to Polio is a cause and effect, or is it a casual correlation? I cannot say for sure. But certainly Dr. Sandler's observations combined with the North Carolina health data from 1949 and 1950 create a powerful theory that, in the name of science and humanity, should absolutely be investigated further.

If you feel you must vaccinate, the Weston A. Price Foundation recommends you take the following precautions:

- ⅄ Wait until the child is at least 2 years old
- ⅄ Do not give more than one vaccination at a time.
- ⅄ Never vaccinate when the child is sick
- ⅄ Be sure that the vaccines are thimerosal-free
- ⅄ Supplement the child with extra cod liver oil, vitamin C, and B12 before each shot
- ⅄ Obtain a medical exemption if the child has had a bad reaction to a vaccination before or if there is a personal or family history of vaccine reactions, convulsions or neurological disorders, severe allergies and/or immune system disorders

I would also suggest supplementing with the amino acid glutathione several days before and after vaccines are administered. Glutathione is a powerful antioxidant that can help the liver clear toxins.

Opting-Out … so far, we still have the right to choose. As of 2011, all 50 states have enacted vaccine laws that require proof children have received certain vaccines in order to attend day-care, middle school, high school and college.

However, in most states citizens currently have the legal right to opt-out of using vaccines. All 50 states allow a medical exemption to vaccination (medical exemptions must be approved by an MD or DO), 48 states allow a religious exemption to vaccination; and 18 states allow a personal, philosophical or conscientious belief exemption to vaccination. However medical exemptions are becoming increasingly difficult to obtain and enforce as many large institutions refuse to respect the opinion of the doctor writing them. There are cases where MDs have written medical exemptions stating that their patient has a prior history of adverse reactions to a vaccine, yet the patients involved were still told that they were required to be vaccinated. Large institutions like hospitals and medical schools often believe they know better than individuals and still require the vaccine for employment or admission, even in cases where the individual people involved had prior adverse reactions.

Vaccine exemptions are constantly under attack in every state because the Big Pharma/Medical Industry lobby is trying to take them away, especially the religious and philosophical or conscientious belief exemptions.

I would never advocate any law that takes away someone's right *to use or refuse* vaccinations. Especially given that there is so little actual clean science about vaccine effectiveness, all options need to be legally protected for everyone.

Part 5: Conclusion

Parents who decide against vaccinating their children are often called thoughtless. In my experience, however, the vast majority of parents who consciously choose to opt-out of vaccination protocols have given the matter a great deal of thought – far more in fact, than the vast majority of parents who simply tell their kids to roll up their sleeves and stick out their arms the day their doctor says it's vaccine time. There is a lot to think about. Most vaccines were not the true cause of substantial declines in disease rates in the late 1800s through the first half of the 20th century. Enhanced sanitation, especially the simple practices of doctors washing their hands between patients and municipalities sanitizing drinking water, should be given the lion's share of the credit for substantially reducing infectious diseases during that time span.

All vaccines can produce minor or major side-effects, including death, and the long-term effects of all vaccines are unknown (especially when considering the large number of doses and combinations typically administered today). The effectiveness, extent of the unwanted side-effects, and long-term effects of vaccines may never be known because those in control say it would be unethical to do scientific double blind testing. They claim it would be unethical to knowingly deprive people in the control (placebo) group the "benefits" of vaccines. It would be relatively easy to to compare the health and well-being of vaccinated versus unvaccinated populations using those who choose to *willingly* opt-out as the unvaccinated group. Amish children or many chiropractor's children could be included and studied in the unvaccinated group. Obviously that would not provide a perfect comparison because vaccination would not be an isolated variable. However, it could be a way to begin a thought-provoking and constructive discussion.

In the US, when reports come out about a few cases of whooping cough, measles, or other diseases, it is often not definitively reported whether or not the affected kids had been vaccinated. Why? That information could be very helpful but it doesn't seem that public health officials want us to have it.

Rather than share straight talk about whether or not a sick kid has been vaccinated, health officials often use the term, *unknown status*. I don't accept that as a good-faith effort to find the truth. My family was once the target of a health department vaccination investigation and I can tell you with certainty, that when health officials really want to know vaccination status, they find out, quickly and definitively.

Vaccine makers already have 95% of the market sewn up. If they did scientific safety and effectiveness studies with the hopes of capturing the last 5%, and if those studies ended up proving that vaccines were unsafe or ineffective, it would be devastating to their bottom line. Unfortunately, that's why we'll never see truly scientific studies. Vaccine makers don't want to take the chance of upsetting their balance sheets.

US government oversight agencies have made it their policy to blindly accept everything Big Pharma claims to be true about vaccine safety and effectiveness. Before you choose whether or not to vaccinate yourself or your child, a mature, thinking person should do a logical, benefit to risk assessment. Most pediatricians or family practitioners don't do their own primary research so they are not equipped to help you much here. They usually simply parrot drug company propaganda.

What are the scientifically proven, likely or possible benefits of vaccination compared to the scientifically proven, likely or possible side effects? To find out, you will need to educate yourself. The following books and websites can provide a thought provoking counterpoint to the predictable mainstream medical information produced by Big Pharma that your doctor will invariably provide.

Resources for more vaccine information:

The National Vaccine Information Center (NVIC), http://www.nvic.org/

Dr. Mercola's Vaccine Website http://vaccines.mercola.com/

Dr. Mercola is one of the most prolific forces in the United States for disseminating truthful information about virtually all aspects of natural healthcare.

Dissolving Illusions: Disease, Vaccines, and the Forgotten History authors Roman Bystrianyk and Suzanne Humphries MD, offer 160 year's worth of historically significant public health data to help you get an accurate picture of vaccine effectiveness.

Vaccines, Are they Really Safe & Effective? By Neil Miller

What About Immunizations? Exposing the Vaccine Philosophy by Cynthia Cournoyer

Saying No To Vaccines by Sherri Tenpenny, D.O.

25

The Missing Link In The Immune System

Learn How Probiotics Help Keep You Healthy

In the last 150 years modern science has provided only two really big breakthroughs in the field of human wellness. In the 1860s doctors figured out that washing their hands between patients would help prevent the spread of infection. Around 1905, municipalities began disinfecting drinking water. The evidence is clear that these two advancements are overwhelmingly responsible for the vast reduction of most widespread infectious diseases.

When it comes to taking personal responsibility for our health, we should understand an important point that doctors seldom publicize: **Abundant beneficial bacteria found in the soil (see chapter four) and the gut, are essential for all aspects of optimum health, despite our culture's microbe-phobia.**

We've all heard of people who are prescribed antibiotics from their doctor and for months thereafter catch every bug that goes around. This occurs because the antibiotics indiscriminately kill all bacteria, good and bad, thereby disrupting an important part of our natural defenses. Digestion and immunity problems after using antibiotics can usually be averted by ingesting premium probiotics (probiotics are microorganisms that offer some form of health benefit to the host) to re-seed the gut with essential beneficial bacteria following antibiotic use. Probiotics can come from traditionally fermented foods or in the form of capsules or liquids purchased from a health food store.

The 60 trillion beneficial bacteria that reside deep in a healthy human gastrointestinal tract, help prevent invading pathogens from ever reaching our bloodstream. They create a living shield that inhibits pathogens including E. coli, salmonella, unhealthy yeasts, and other threats, from penetrating the intestinal lining and reaching the bloodstream. These friendly bacteria also help manufacture essential nutrients like vitamins B-12, K-2, as well as many immune enhancing compounds that scientists have yet to understand or even fully identify. Further, good bacteria play a vital role in the digestive process by breaking down food so it can be absorbed through the intestinal wall.

Bacteria in the soil help break down nutrients so plants can better absorb them and stay nourished and healthy. In our gut, beneficial bacteria complete the digestion of food so nutrients can pass through the intestinal wall, helping to keep us nourished and healthy. From the bacteria in live, healthy soil, to the beneficial bacteria in the human digestive tract, these microorganisms play a never-ending fundamental role in the transformation and assimilation of life-sustaining nutrients.

The people of every major culture on earth have had some kind of fermented food in their regular daily diet providing

them with good bacteria and enzymes – all people except those in the modern North American culture. We've all heard of popular time-tested fermented foods like sauerkraut, miso, kim-chee, yogurt, and kefir. Ancient Rome had a fermented fish sauce called liquamen and ancient China had its own, tart tasting, fermented sauce that's credited with being the original "ketchup." In years past pickles, relishes and other condiments were natural, unpasteurized and actually provided beneficial bacteria and enzymes. They were held in high esteem for their health enhancing properties. Unfortunately, virtually all commercially available mass-market pickles and condiments in the US are now highly processed and provide few, if any, health benefits.

The National Cancer Center Research Institute of Japan, confirmed in the journal <u>Carcinogenesis</u>, that an abundance of cancer preventing nutrients are found in traditional fermented soy foods such as miso, tempeh, natto, and fermented soy milk – qualities almost completely absent in unfermented soy foods. In addition, miso, tempeh, and especially natto, convey proven cardio-protective qualities.

Today, in India, approximately 200,000,000 people a day consume a fermented lentil and rice preparation called idli. Idli is so gentle, and its nutrients so easy to digest and bio-available, that it's regularly used in hospitals to sustain the sick and the very young.

Dr. Weil has stated: "Probiotics are an effective treatment for diarrhea, lactose intolerance, irritable bowel syndrome, vaginal yeast infections, oral thrush, Crohn's disease, and ulcerative colitis. When there's a family history of allergy or eczema, babies receiving probiotics in their first six months of life (and whose mothers took probiotics during the last trimester of pregnancy) are less prone to eczema. Children with autism can also benefit from probiotics, possibly because probiotics can help decrease leakage (into the bloodstream) of large molecules from the gut that can trigger immune reactions that have effects on brain function." Probiotics have also been shown to be effective treating women with recurring urinary tract infections who suffer from burning during urination.

Groundbreaking work linking intellect and emotion to gut health is being done by Dr. Natasha Campbell-McBride. Dr. Campbell-McBride runs the Cambridge Nutrition Clinic in the UK and is recognized as one of the world's leading experts in treating children and adults with learning disabilities, autism and other mental disorders, as well as children and adults with digestive and immune disorders.

Her book: Gut and Psychology Syndrome (GAPS): Natural Treatment Of Autism, ADHD, Dyslexia, Dyspraxia, Depression and Schizophrenia, explores the connection between the patient's physical state, especially intestinal health, and their brain function. Campbell-McBride explains how toxicity in the gut can flow throughout the body and into the brain, where it can cause symptoms of autism, ADHD, dyslexia, dyspraxia, depression, schizophrenia and other disorders.

Life changing case studies from patients following the GAPS Diet protocol at her clinic have earned Campbell-McBride international accolades. Her solutions are revolutionary, yet steeped in time-tested wisdom. Campbell-McBride's primary tool for rehabilitating an unhealthy gut is prescribing naturally fermented foods and probiotic supplements to create a healthy balance of intestinal flora in her patients.

The comprehensive and brilliant book by Sandor Katz titled: <u>The Art of Fermentation</u> can teach you how to make traditional, ultra-healthy, naturally fermented foods in your own kitchen.

For thousands of years, our bodies' exposure to a biologically diverse assortment of bacteria has kept our immune systems in *fighting shape,* ready to defend us against all challengers. Nonetheless, our culture has bought the idea that we should be terrified of germs and obsessed with hygiene. Every new sensationalized report of the latest killer microbe creates fear of interaction with all forms of microscopic life. The manufacturers of anti-bacterial soaps have done a good job for themselves by monetizing those fears. But, are fewer people catching colds and flus since these antibacterial soaps have become popular? The evidence does not suggest this. In addition, antibiotic-resistant infections such as MRSA (Methicillin-resistant Staphylococcus aureus) are on the rise.

The immune system educates and adapts itself from direct experience. The "hygiene hypothesis" attributes the dramatic increase in asthma and allergies to a lack of exposure to microorganisms found in healthy soil; in other words – insufficient education at the microscopic level. Dr. David Rosenstreich, director of Allergy and Immunology at Albert Einstein Medical School in New York stated: "The cleaner we live ... the more likely we'll get asthma and allergies."

A tree grows from soil nutrients. After its natural lifespan, it falls to the forest floor and would remain there forever unless bacteria worked to break it down. Fortunately in nature,

bacteria will act, and the tree will be absorbed back into the soil and become soil nutrients again. From there it will support new growth. This is the cycle of life and beneficial bacteria play a vital and irreplaceable role both in the soil and the gut.

26

Healthy Pets Help Make
Happy Families

The Shocking Truth About Pet Foods

When our entire family is healthy, happy, and energetic, our world becomes a brighter place. For the nearly 65% of the American households who consider their pet a family member, the health and happiness of pets plays an important role in family well-being.

With annual routine vet bills averaging around $100 and dog or cat surgery often costing thousands of dollars, plus extras for X-rays and prescription medications, it also makes financial sense to keep our pets healthy.

Our German-born Rottweiler, Max, was the 120-pound family pet my kids grew up with (a cute little doggie he was). Max was still happy and energetic at age 14, while most of his Rottweiler buddies had died from cancers at seven or eight. He went to a vet only once his life. Good nutrition played a huge role in keeping him happy and healthy.

Just like for their human owners, clean, high quality food plays a critical role in pet health. However, cutting through the slick marketing and selecting healthy food for your pet requires a little education.

The sad truth about most mainstream pet food brands is not pretty. Foods that are deemed unfit for humans are often intentionally used in pet food manufacturing. These unsavory ingredients can lawfully make it into pet foods, and may include: road kill, slaughterhouse waste, deceased animals (no matter what the cause of death), spoiled supermarket foods (sometimes with the packaging intact), and even euthanized pets (most often euthanized with toxic chemicals).

Choosing healthy pet foods is not as easy as looking for the words premium or natural. **Unlike the term "organic," the words "premium" and "natural" are completely unregulated by the United States Department of Agriculture (USDA).** While some companies can rightfully stand by claims of being "all-natural" the sad truth is that most are simply preying on well-intentioned consumers. Not to say you cannot purchase quality products with "natural" or "premium" on the label, but don't buy them *solely because* these terms appear on the label.

To avoid choosing a dog food that might contain horrific ingredients, the best way to minimize the risk is to never buy products made with generic animal ingredients. In this case generic means animal based ingredients which do not specify the source animal. They use non-specific words like "meat" or "poultry," rather than the actual species like "beef" or "chicken." According to the pet food industry, meat can come from virtually any kind of mammal. So, unlike beef meal, which must come from beef, generic meat meal can legally be from road kill, dead zoo animals, horses, or dead cats and dogs. In addition, high quality pet foods will always be made from ingredients that are USDA approved for human consumption. Furthermore, just like the standards you have when shopping for human members of your family, you should never buy pet products with artificial colors or preservatives.

The best diet you can feed your dog or cat is a homemade, balanced, raw diet. Understandably, it's fairly costly and time consuming to prepare. A homemade, balanced, cooked diet supplemented with some raw foods would be next best. From a practical perspective, feeding your pet high quality commercially prepared kibble made from ingredients approved for human consumption and adding a homemade "booster mix" should provide your pet with everything they need to stay healthy. It will be reasonably priced and quick to prepare. If you're traveling or squeezed for time, you can always just feed the kibble for short durations and your pet will still be fine.*

You can easily prepare a week's worth of booster mix in about 10 minutes, then just add some every day to your pet's kibble.

Booster Mix Recipe

- ⚔ 2 lbs. of raw ground beef, chicken or turkey **Or substitute** 1 qt. of organic unsweetened yogurt or 8-10 cooked or raw eggs
- ⚔ 1 cup of hemp, flax or fish oil
- ⚔ 1 cup of small diced or flaked seaweed
- ⚔ 1 cup of chopped garlic***

---

* At our store, we've always sold the Solid Gold line of natural pet foods. Customers are usually very impressed with the results.

** Some experts opine that garlic should not be fed to dogs. Advice from Dr. Pitcairn's book is to the contrary. I've always found that garlic seemed good for our pets, possibly providing some measure of flea protection.

- ⅄ 1 bunch of parsley, finely chopped
- ⅄ Mix with food processor or by hand.

Adding approximately one cup (or less for smaller dogs) of booster mix per day to dry kibble will provide your special "family member" with:

- ⅄ **Essential fatty acids** from the oils for healthy skin, coat, eyes and ears.
- ⅄ **Readily absorbable minerals** from the seaweeds for healthy bones and joints
- ⅄ **Parasite & pathogen protection** from the garlic
- ⅄ **Breath enhancement,** enzymes and live vitamin C from the parsley

Frequent use of pet probiotics will boost immunity and improve digestion. In addition, 1/4 to 1/2 teaspoon a day of Spirulina powder has brought back the "pep in their step" of many family pets in their golden years. Your whole family deserves to be healthy all year round. Plus in the long run, healthy pets will save us humans lots of money in vet bills.

Two of the best resources to guide you through the adventure of natural pet care are the books <u>Real Food for Healthy Dogs and Cats</u> by Beth Taylor and Karen Shaw Becker, DVM and <u>Dr. Pitcairn's Guide to Natural Health for Dogs and Cats</u>. These books will arm you with knowledge to cut through the slick marketing tactics of major pet food companies and select the healthy food your pet deserves. Remember, whether human, canine, or feline, clean, high quality food plays a critical role in health.

27

Why The Affordable Care Act (Obamacare) Misses The Mark

How To Fix A Fundamentally Flawed Healthcare System

The Affordable Care Act, or *Obamacare*, was passed into law in 2010 and upheld by the Supreme Court in 2012. This nearly two-thousand page law has its share of complexities. It has been, to say the least, polarizing; but the truth about our new healthcare act likely settles somewhere between Fox News' right-wing, unrelenting criticism and MSNBC's left-wing, unabashed praise. **In my opinion there are fundamental shortcomings that this "Healthcare Reform" act completely fails to address that nearly nobody is talking about.**

There are exceptions to many sections of Obamacare but the main features of the Affordable Care Act are:

⅄ The law requires all Americans to have health insurance by 2014 or pay a tax penalty

⅄ Insurance can be purchased through your state's Health Insurance Marketplace Exchange

⅄ Insurance companies cannot drop you when you are sick or for making a mistake on your application

⅄ You cannot be denied coverage for pre-existing conditions

⅄ Subsidies will be available for low income individuals and families

According to CNN, 60% of all personal bankruptcies are due to medical expenses. Most who filed for bankruptcy protection were middle-class, well-educated homeowners. Obamacare should, theoretically, eliminate both lifetime and annual insurance pay-out limits. This should help protect many Americans from going bankrupt and allow them to continue treatment as long as they need it, not just until their dollar or time limit has been reached.

I can see benefits to some of these features. However, the biggest criticism I have about our new national healthcare law is that it does little to discuss or promote actual health and wellness. In the interest of well-being, sustainability and affordability, first and foremost Americans need to be taught as much about their own health as their doctors know about drugs and disease.. **As it is currently configured, the American "Healthcare" system is not really about health at all ... it**

The Vision Of A Genius

"The doctor of the future will give no medication, but will interest his patients in the care of the human frame, diet, and in the cause and prevention of disease."
– Thomas Edison ...1898

232

would be more accurate to label it: the American *Disease-care* system.

The Affordable Care Act focuses primarily on how people will pay for sickness treatments that rely on obscenely expensive, toxic pharmaceuticals and surgeries as primary healing modalities. However, the discussion about people's ability to pay for these treatments distracts from the much bigger issue, which is: What is the true value (or lack thereof) of many of these modern drugs and treatments?

Former American Medical Association chairman Raymond Scalettar came right out and said: "One-half to one-third of the $2.2 trillion per year America spends on healthcare is simply unnecessary." Why is that?

One simple reason is inefficiency created by a staggering bureaucracy. Duke University Hospital provides a typical example. It has 900 hospital beds and 1,300 billing clerks! What those clerks are doing in US hospitals is using different systems to figure out how to bill different insurers. Large hospitals in countries with single-payer systems will only have a handful of billing clerks. That is not saying single-payer systems are better, but they do have fewer administrative costs and in that aspect clearly waste less money.

No discussion about medical inefficiency would be complete without considering the thoughts of Dr. Arnold Relman. Dr. Relman was the editor of the *New England Journal of Medicine* for 23 years. He was also president of The American Federation of Clinical Research, the American Society of Clinical Investigation, and The Association of American Physicians – the only person to hold all four positions.

In a thought provoking article he wrote in 1980, Relman impugned the American healthcare system for being motivated more by monetary profits than healing the sick. One of Relman's suggested remedies to more efficiently deliver medical services was a single (tax-payer) supported medical insurance system (like Medicare) to replace myriad private insurance companies, which he referred to as "parasites."

I believe another primary reason hundreds of billions of dollars spent on healthcare in America is being wasted is that, in essence, mainstream medical schools enable Big Pharma to teach medical students about expensive patented drugs, *not* about actual health.

A study done by the American Medical Student Association (AMSA) showed that only 4 of 158 medical schools in the US banned drug company representatives from their campuses: The University of South Dakota's

Who Is Big Pharma?

In 2012, the top 10 pharmaceutical companies (by sales) were:

Johnson & Johnson	$67.2 billion
Pfizer	$58.9 billion
Novartis	$56.7 billion
Roche	$47.8 billion
Merck	$47.3 billion
Sanofi	$46.4 billion
GlaxoSmithKline	$39.9 billion
Abbot Labratories/AbbVie	$39.9 billion
AstraZeneca	$28.0 billion
Bayer HealthCare	$24.3 billion

Sanford School of Medicine, Florida State University College of Medicine, Stony Brook University School of Medicine, New York, and the Commonwealth Medical College, Scranton PA., all received perfect scores in that area.

The group also discovered that one Harvard professor, who promoted the benefits of cholesterol reducing statin drugs to his students, was a paid consultant for 10 drug companies, including five makers of the cholesterol drugs he enthusiastically promoted.

The study uncovered more obvious conflicts of interests involved in the shaping of medical students' beliefs. In 2008 alone, drug companies gave more than $11.5 million to Harvard for medical research and education. Overall, Harvard Medical School received an "F" – the worst possible grade – from AMSA, which ranks 150 medical schools according to their ties to the pharmaceutical industry. At the University of Oklahoma Health Sciences Center about 13.5% of the budget came from industrial-pharmaceutical sources in 2003. Drug giants AstraZeneca, Merck, Novartis and Upjohn all made large "contributions" to the budget. There were 183 industrial-pharmaceutical grants in that one school alone, that year totaling $13.8 million. Similar scenarios are in play at virtually all major medical schools.

Obamacare does nothing to stop drug companies from essentially buying influence at medical schools, thereby shaping the beliefs and paradigms that students will be pressured into adopting; nor does it change the fact that typical medical school curricula fail to include classes in wellness and disease prevention. **In essence, Harvard and other medical schools act**

as business agents who help drug manufacturers choose and train their de-facto sales force (the graduating doctors).

Further, our new national healthcare law does nothing to address the fact that over 4 billion prescriptions were written for drugs in America in 2011 - an average of over 13 for each man, woman and child, while the average senior citizen is prescribed 28 per year. The profit made when selling these prescriptions is basically the return on investment (ROI) for the money the pharmaceutical companies "donate" to the medical schools by paying tens of millions for all that "unbiased" research. If all these prescriptions drugs could successfully treat and cure disease, the United States would have the healthiest and longest lived inhabitants on the planet. Sadly, they don't and we're not.

Marcia Angell, MD, former editor in chief of the *New England Journal of Medicine*, one of the world's most well respected medical journals said the pharmaceutical industry "has moved very far from it's original high purpose of discovering and producing useful new drugs. Now primarily a marketing machine to sell drugs of dubious benefit, this industry uses its wealth and power to co-opt every institution that might stand in its way, including the US congress, Food and Drug Administration, academic medical centers, and the medical profession itself."

Nationally recognized healthcare educator Dr. Archelle Georgiou says that relying on doctors may actually shorten your lifespan. She has studied many isolated communities around the world whose inhabitants live longer, healthier lives than the greater populace. In the following examples their excellent diet, exercise, stress management, sleep patterns, recreation, farming/gardening and emotional support systems are all ***naturally integrated*** aspects of their traditional lifestyles – not willful, dutiful adjuncts patched onto crazy, stress-filled, store-bought lives. Some examples are:

⅄ The Greek island of Ikaria, where inhabitants are over four times more likely to live to age 90 than Americans are and they suffer less depression and about a quarter the rate of dementia - **yet there is virtually no healthcare infrastructure.** Their traditional foods, beverages, and herbal preparations are locally grown and prepared. They care little there about precise clock-time.

⅄ The remote Nicoya peninsula in Costa Rica where a man at age 60 has about twice the chance of reaching age 90 than a man living in the US - again, with virtually no healthcare infrastructure.

⅄ Sardinia is an island 120 miles off the coast of Italy where the people - mostly farmers and shepherds - are particularly long-lived. In fact, just one town of 1,700 people, Ovodda, boasts five centenarians. Some of the explanation for Sardinians' longevity may be genetic, but it's also likely much of the credit should go to their diet. They eat a healthy Mediterranean diet, that includes consuming lots of locally grown and produced foods including raw milk and cheese from grass-fed goats. They are known for walking a lot and maintaining a positive attitude and sense of humor about life.

⅄ Okinawa - a chain of islands 360 miles off the coast of Japan - has the world's highest prevalence of proven centenarians: 740 out of a population of 1.3 million. **Okinawan seniors**

not only have the highest life expectancy in the world, but also the highest health expectancy: they remain vigorous and healthy into old age, suffering relatively few age-related ailments. Widespread gardening provides an opportunity for exercise, sunlight, and nutritious food. Okinawans also follow an old adage that says "eat until you are 80% full" instead of gorging (American style all-you-can-eat buffets might not be a big hit there).

The lifestyle followed in all of these cultures continues to naturally include the time-tested four pillars of health referred to in chapter one. If Big Pharma could patent, bottle, sell, and profit from the healthy traditions embedded in these cultures, you can be sure there would be classes taught about them at every major medical school in the US.

So far, the intense national healthcare debate in the US still has not included serious dialog about health. The "healthcare" debate has focused primarily on ensuring that people don't go bankrupt paying absurd prices for drugs and treatments, rather than the quality of the healthcare itself. We need comprehensive definitions of the words "health" and "care" before our total well-being will be served.

Obamacare does provide ways for average folks to pay for obscenely expensive medical treatments but it needs to go further. Most doctors' business models have them operating under narrow time constraints in a staggering bureaucracy. The debt many incur paying for medical school puts them under even greater stress after graduation to simply put their "noses to the grindstone" and start producing. Over 85% of medical students graduate with student debt in the range of $150,000 - $200,000, and that doesn't include costs for undergrad work. For doctors, there is no real money and little repeat business in empowering their patients to be less dependent on them. Even if young doctors acknowledge the problem and conflicting interests in play, their goal is, understandably, to start immediately earning for their families, not to repair a broken medical system.

In some countries, medical school is free to students who are willing to assist under-served communities for several years after graduation at a reasonable wage. Not only has Cuba provided such training to thousands of specialists from the Caribbean, Latin America, and Africa, but more recently, they even offered this training to US students. In July 2007, eight US students graduated and 88 more enrolled. The first to graduate, Cedric Edwards, is now working at Montefiore Hospital in New York City's Bronx borough. Removing the pressure of paying back student loans may allow doctors the freedom to think outside the box, with far less regard for monetary gain and more emphasis on overall patient well-being.

Dr. Andrew Weil has stated that while more medical research is important, at this point it's not at the top of the list of factors needed for improving the healthcare system. He places teaching doctors and medical students the concepts of Integrative Medicine as a far more urgent need.

If we continue to allow the drug manufacturers and their supporters at the FDA, physician trade organizations such as the American Medical Association, and insurance companies to frame these discussions, we will undoubtedly receive

"affordable" healthcare that's expensive, toxic, habit forming, and ultimately nothing I would recommend you regularly entrust your health to.

Real national healthcare reform would actively encourage a change from relying on invasive, extremely expensive, profit driven, high risk treatments like drugs and surgeries to time-tested, low-cost, natural methods of optimizing health and wellness.

28

Conclusion: Critical Thinking Is Your Best Medicine

Making Good Decisions Is Nature's Universal Healthcare Plan

Making health decisions based on holistic thinking that has proven to be sensible since man first walked the planet, is the most far-reaching way to stay healthy. Using your body in the way it was designed, has always been, is now, and always will be, the best way to pay the "premium" for true, universal healthcare. For that reason, optimum health can often begin by saying "No" to your doctor.

Another crucial step to improving your health and well-being is to strengthen your resistance against the onslaught of drug company advertising that will go to almost any lengths to convince you to be a lifetime customer for their toxic drugs. **Getting your thinking straight should be *priority-one* on the path to lasting health.**

During cold and flu season, everyone is trying to optimize their immune systems. In chapter 22, I suggested that **the easiest way to win the "cold war" is to understand and then change** the **"battlefield" conditions.** Factors that will keep you healthy are generally the exact opposite of the factors that support proliferation of cold and flu viruses. Keeping your bloodstream slightly alkaline by getting sufficient deep sleep, avoiding excess sugar and alcohol and fueling your body with abundant healthful nutrients are three of the basics offered in that chapter.

When addressing long term survival from life threatening illnesses like cancer, patients and their doctors typically focus first on mounting a bio-chemical assault on the offending disease. However, **using this strategy alone does not engage the most powerful part of the patients' immune system; their brain!** When I am asked, "what's the best cancer treatment?" the advice I offer in chapter 20 is for people to thoroughly research the available options and then choose the ones that *they* personally feel most confident about. **Carefully studying, making your own informed choice, and moving forward with confidence, is going to provide the best chance for long-term wellness.**

When a bachelor opens the Tupperware container from the back of his fridge with the 3-week old, pungent smelling, fur-covered leftovers, he has two choices: eat it, or throw it out. At a minimum, his short-term health hangs in the balance. Will his white blood cells, antibodies, bone marrow or other parts of his immune system help make the decision? **No, his brain alone, deciding whether to eat it or skip it, is the only thing protecting him from certain illness at that moment.**

Every chapter in this book has focused on stimulating and strengthening this most basic and powerful part of your body's defenses. In chapter 18, where the potential health dangers of cell phones are discussed, I pointed out that it took 70 years for the asbestos industry to *come-clean* about the carcinogenic nature of their products. My point was to demonstrate that just because a product has decades of strong sales, doesn't mean that the product is truly safe and will ultimately stand the test of time. **Profitability and popularity are not proof of safety.**

Even though the cell phone industry issues assurances that their products are *completely* safe, the 2014 Bordeaux University study supported other international studies, suggesting a higher threat of brain tumors observed among heavier cell phone users. Using a cellphone for more than half an hour a day over five years can triple the risk of developing certain types of brain cancer, compared with those who used their phone rarely. The risk is highest for Ipsilateral exposure. (Ipsilateral exposure refers to cell phone use on the same side of the head most or all of the time). **To protect yourself from serious health hazards of cell phones, be smart and keep the cell phone away from your head.** Use it as a speakerphone or avoid long conversations with the phone pressed against your head, even one inch away can make a big difference. If you do need to hold the phone against your head for some period of time, it is important to switch ears, so that the phone does not rest on the same side of your head all the time. **Your brain needs to remember to take these precautions.**

In the case of smoking, the (in)famous TV and magazine ads from the 1950s boasted: "More doctors smoke Camels than any other brand." Those ads were based on surveys of over 100,000 medical doctors. However, by 1965 the Surgeon General had determined that no matter who smoked them, cigarettes caused cancer. So, just because a doctor or, in the case of cigarettes, even a future president (Ronald Reagan was in many of the ads), endorses a product, that doesn't mean it is a healthy, smart choice. To protect yourself from smoking you don't need antioxidants, vitamins or more T-cells. The only part of your "immune system" **you need to engage is your brain, by simply making the decision not to smoke.** There can be no greater defeat for every part of your immune system than death.

In chapter 23, I wrote about natural childbirth and baby care. The Cesarean birth rate in the US is now over 30% and doctors routinely advise 35 doses of different vaccines for babies in their first 15 months of life. Despite those "advancements," **the US currently ranks 50th in the world in infant mortality.** That means 49 other countries do a better job of keeping babies alive. And the US maternal mortality rate has increased 50% in the past 25 years. Something is very wrong with these pictures.

If we use our brains to think about it, maybe there are better ways to help insure the health of babies and their mothers than following what has now become the US medical model. Remember back in the 50s, part of that model included doctors recommending that newborns not be breastfed. Fortunately, the American Academy of Pediatrics now recommends breastfeeding for the first 12 months of life. **Thanks to more enlightened thinking on this subject, we've returned to a time-tested, biologically perfect, tradition.**

Whether it's choosing the most nutritious food, finding healthy alternatives to prescription drugs, increasing the survival rate of babies, avoiding unnecessary cancer risks from modern inventions, or preventing osteoporosis and heart attack, **thinking for yourself and using your brain to make good decisions will provide more protection from sickness, disease, and death than anything else you can do, no matter what the cost.**

Seeking the truth about health issues can sometimes feel like David battling Goliath. I understand that it's not always easy - otherwise everyone would do it. Big Pharma checkbooks regularly shape "independent" research to an alarming degree. For example, in 2008 alone, drug companies gave more than $11.5 million to Harvard for medical research and education. Time magazine reported: "Of Harvard's 8,900 professors and lecturers, 1,600 admit that either they or a family member have had some kind of business link to drug companies - sometimes worth hundreds of thousands of dollars - that could bias their teaching or research." Columbia University received nearly $790 million from licensing agreements with bio-tech and pharmaceutical companies during the 17-year life of its medical school's bio-synthesis patent, according to drugwatch.com. These are startling revelations! Do you think there might be a reason to question the limited curricula presented to med students, or the conclusions that are published by some of our top teaching and research institutions, given their cozy connection to Big Pharma?

Similar funding models are repeated at virtually every major medical school in the US. Well meaning, open minded medical students have nearly no chance of leaving that environment with their diplomas unless they learn to salute and recite the answers that have been bought and paid for by drug company giants like: AstraZeneca, Merck, Novartis, Pfizer, and others (Big Pharma).

According to the World Health Organization, the US has by far the highest per capita use of conventional (toxic) medicines in the world. Americans use over 40% of all the drugs manufactured worldwide annually. However, the US ranks only forty-second in life expectancy. Clearly, there are more effective ways

to maintain and improve health than turning to Big Pharma for advice. Becoming your own health expert by accessing unbiased health information and thinking independently is the best way to elevate yourself and your family to the level of wellness you were born to enjoy. Please remember that making good decisions is the cornerstone of Nature's Universal Healthcare Plan.

29

Natural Healing Success Stories

The "Hippocrates Seal Of Approval"

After finishing the first 28 chapters in this book, I was encouraged by Dr. Janet Levatin (author of this book's foreword), to add a chapter that included a representative sample of some of the health success stories our customers have shared over the years. She pointed out that even though a successful natural healing story is just one individual account, for the person who experienced it, it's 100% real and if we get thousands of similar stories on one subject (gluten intolerance or vaccine complications, as examples), that becomes a body of evidence unto itself. **Significant anecdotal evidence can help provide clear direction for institutions or individual scientists when they choose areas to investigate.**

**Dr. Andrew Weil On Health
Success Stories and Anecdotes:**

"Most medical scientists tend to drop all testimonials into wastebaskets labeled, Anecdotal Evidence. In medical usage, "anecdotal evidence" tends to mean "of no scientific value or importance." I take a different view of this material and am interested in why so many doctors have a hard time with it ... it's foolish to ignore testimonial evidence because it may suggest directions for experimental inquiry as well as provide clues to the nature of healing ... The essence of good science is open minded inquiry, so would it not make sense to try, at least, to verify the stories? ... Science is the orderly gathering of knowledge by methodical inquiry and experiment, but where do you get ideas to inquire about or experiment with except through your experience with the world around you?"

I completely agree with Drs. Weil and Levatin and while one or even several anecdotes on a given subject are seldom enough justification to steadfastly adhere to a definite opinion, totally ignoring all anecdotal evidence is more than anything else, a symptom of a closed, dead, mind. Many doctors (maybe even your doctor) might be quick to dismiss the following natural health success stories as nothing more than meaningless, isolated anecdotes. If my doctor insisted on remaining attached to that mentality, I would fire him/her and find another who has a functionally younger and more inquisitive mind.

If Big Pharma, through its influence at medical schools, can keep the public and doctors convinced that the *only* legitimate and valid health outcome information comes from formal studies that are often extremely expensive and difficult to conduct and publish, the drug companies can make sure that only rich and powerful institutions and corporations are in a position to control what gets validated.

It would be far better for humankind and the environment if the health paradigm driving research was actually focused on sustainable health instead of corporate profits, but very often it is not.

Listening to individual health success stories or healing anecdotes can be very useful. I read and study quite a bit. But when a customer has a specific health challenge, *they* are the ones who study *that* specific subject the hardest and are most likely to find a solution. No one is more motivated to find relief than the person (or their family) who is suffering.

Customers in my health food store often share with me their stories about using healing methods and dietary supplements that mainstream doctors seldom suggest. From them, I often see and hear very credible (often verified by doctors' lab tests) anecdotes of cholesterol reductions, bone density increases, blood pressure reductions, vision improvements, relief from enlarged prostate symptoms, improved sleep, lower stress and overall improved heath in many other areas.

In conveying the following natural healing success stories, I intentionally omitted the brand names of specific products because my purpose here is not to sell merchandise, but rather to offer examples of what is possible through simple, natural methods. One of the most profound anecdotes, a cancer remission story that was basically free (zero cost), appears at the end of chapter 20.

Three Heart Disease Recovery Stories

1) When Don was admitted to the hospital in June of 2000, he was in bad shape. He was told his heart was enlarged to nearly four times its normal size. He needed oxygen continuously and was not able to walk the short distance from the hospital bed to the bathroom. The prognosis from his cardiologist was bleak: congestive heart failure with 2-4 weeks to live.

Purely by chance, Don's daughter, a dialysis nurse, was treating a retired cardiologist and she mentioned her dad's story. Her patient said one thing: "Get your dad Co-Q-10." Don's family came to our store and left with a bottle of 150 mg capsules of Co-enzyme Q10, a nutrient

My Observation

I've learned over the years that what a doctor really means when he/she says you have x-amount of time to live is: Based on what they've seen or been taught about a condition like yours, if you follow their advice, there's an excellent chance you will die in the time frame they predicted.

If you want to live longer than they predicted, you would be wise to try an alternative to their advice.

Don's case is an excellent example

all your cells require to process oxygen for energy. He began using 2-a-day.

A year later Don was in great spirits, mowing his lawn and feeding his chickens. The local cardiologist who had originally predicted Don would die within two weeks now called him a 74 year-old "miracle boy." Rather than a miracle, I think it was the Co-Q-10.

2) With his permission, we publicized Don's story in the store's newsletter. This was very fortunate for a 77 year-old retired nurse named Barbara. Barbara had a history of declining heart health. including valve and fibrillation problems. A pacemaker helped some, but she was still virtually bedridden. In March of 2004 she was admitted to the hospital and diagnosed with congestive heart failure. Barbara's heart was twice normal size and her ejection fraction was 29% (a measurement under 40 may be evidence of heart failure or cardiomyopathy).

She tried more prescription medications, but unlivable side-effects forced her to quickly discontinue their use. With help, Barbara came to our store where she was told about Don's success story and shown Co-Q-10 and hawthorn berry extract. She began taking 200 mg of Co-Q-10 once per day along with 300 mg of hawthorn extract twice daily and began feeling better within days. Two months later after analyzing her test results, Barb's doctors told her that her heart was much improved and that unless she had more trouble, she should come back in year.

After being bedridden in early March, Barbara walked the mile from her house to our store just four months later to say "thank you!"

An interesting part of this story was that Barbara never told her doctors she was using natural supplements. She was afraid they would refuse to see her if she told them she was using anything other than what they had originally wanted her to use. She is not alone with that fear. It's not uncommon for some of our customers to avoid telling their doctors they have even visited a health food store.

3) Molly and Bill had been married over 60 years. At 90 years-old, Bill still did much of the outdoor work it took to maintain their property. At 89, Molly tried to keep up with shopping, cooking and keeping the house as she always had.

Molly's energy levels had been dropping for years and her doctor told her that her heart was not in good shape. She became easily exhausted in the middle of routine tasks. It got to the point that one day while grocery shopping she became so tired she had to sit down on the floor to rest in the aisle at the supermarket. After that, according to Bill, Molly increasingly spent her time at home in an easy chair with her feet up.

Then they heard one of our radio commercials about the help Co-Q-10 had provided to others. Bill came in and purchased Co-Q-10 and hawthorn berry extract for his wife. About six weeks later, on a cold, snowy day Bill walked into the store with a woman he introduced as his wife Molly. They had been out the previous night dancing to celebrate their wedding anniversary and came to our store to say "thank you."

Even though these stories are essentially individual anecdotes, at some point we should at least be able to suggest we are observing a pattern. Maybe if we include the following we can.

Internationally there have been at least nine placebo-controlled studies on the treatment of heart disease with Co-Q-10. Two each, in the US, Japan, Italy, and Germany, and one in Sweden. There have been at least eight international conferences on the biomedical and clinical aspects of Co-Q-10. Over 3000 papers presented by 200 different physicians and scientists from 18 countries.

Most of the studies focused on the treatment of heart disease and are remarkably consistent. The conclusion: Heart function is significantly improved with Co-Q-10 while producing virtually no adverse side-effects or drug interactions.

Why didn't Don's, Barbara's or Molly's doctors suggest they try Co-Q-10? Maybe because they weren't taught anything about Co-Q-10 in medical school. In Don's case, his doctor's lack of experience nearly proved fatal.

The question I would have for Don's doctor: The next time you see a similar case, will you again tell your patient he has 2-4 weeks to live, or will you at least entertain the possibility that there may be a life-enhancing natural alternative? I believe the answer to that question would clarify whether his cardiologist is motivated more by serving humanity or being a dutiful servant of Big Pharma.

Four Success Stories with One Common Theme

About ten years ago a woman came into our store looking for a specific product that I hadn't heard of. She tried to convince me to carry it, but I was reluctant to risk buying an entire case of a product that I knew nothing about and had no demand for, in order to satisfy one customer.

A month later she was back, asking if we had gotten it in yet. The answer was no. At that point, I still had no idea that this persistently positive woman wasn't done with me or my store.

About a week later I received a call from the manufacturer of the product she was looking for. They said that their company had two customers in our town who would purchase the product from our store if we would carry it. They sealed the deal by offering to front me a case (I wouldn't have to pay until it all sold). I agreed, even though I still knew virtually nothing about the product.

When the case of the product came, they had also included an additional bottle marked "Demo." **Having absolutely no preconceived notion about what to expect (if anything), I studied the directions on the bottle, followed them, put eight drops in a glass of water, and drank it.** Within about 15 minutes, I felt noticeably different. That led to me offering samples to others in the following days. Soon thereafter we sold all twelve bottles, paid our bill, and ordered more.

It turns out this product claimed, among other things, to be the world's number one oxygen enhancing supplement – interesting.

The perfect prospect for this product came in one day. A woman using supplemental oxygen provided by a portable oxygen concentrator (POC) told me that contracting pneumonia seven times in five years had damaged her left lung as a result (according to her doctor). Without her machine, her blood oxygen level typically measured around 74 (dangerously low). She bought some of the oxygen enhancing product and after two months using the product her oxygen level measured 94 without the machine. Just as impressive, after using the product for the entire winter, she told me that was the first time in five years she not gotten sick during what is normally considered the cold and flu season.

We publicized that amazing story and a different woman who had been using supplemental oxygen round-the-clock for 15 years, decided to give the same product a try. In about two weeks she was able to discontinue her supplemental oxygen for 5-8 hours at a time.

In short order, we had two more, for a total for four, extremely similar stories. There must be a point where it is reasonable to consider that we were observing another pattern.

We have literally dozens more success stories from customers using that product with the common themes consistently being fast results, markedly increased energy (sometimes after discontinuing supplemental oxygen) and pain reductions.

Some health problems can be complicated and require extensive effort, expertise and testing to solve. However, despite the fact that a doctor may have charged a large fee, ordered elaborate tests, and prescribed medications, the solution is not always complicated. The following are some individual natural health success stories stories from our customers who were led by their doctors to believe they had a problem that was difficult to solve. As you will read, that is not always the case.

In Fact: <u>S</u>ometimes <u>I</u>t's <u>R</u>eally <u>S</u>imple (SIRS)

Acid reflux:

Acid reflux, Gastroesophageal Reflux Disease (GERD), chronic heartburn, or whatever you want to call it, is a very common affliction. We sell natural products targeted to address it. But sometimes, they're not even needed.

A woman came in looking for relief from what her doctor called acid reflux. She had used prescription medications for this problem, on and off, for a decade, but it had always returned. There are well-documented major problems associated with the long-term use of medications that shut down acid production. Without sufficient stomach acid it is not possible for your body to fully and properly absorb many key nutrients such as vitamin B-12 and calcium. That is why the FDA acknowledges that long-term use of these drugs has been linked to increased incidence of hip, wrist, and spine fractures. Long-term use has also been conclusively linked to increased risk of pneumonia and to being more susceptible to food poisoning. It's no wonder she was looking for a way to be able to eat without needing drugs.

I asked a little about her eating habits. My questions brought out the fact that she regularly consumed **ice-cold** drinks with her meals. I gave her the same advice I had written in my monthly health column published in the local newspaper: Drinking ice-cold liquids is one of the worst things you can do for your digestion.

When you really stop and consider it, you realize that everyday, year-round use of ice wasn't even a widely available option until about 75 years ago. Think about the shock that jumping naked into an ice-cold lake causes to the outside of your body – goose bumps, skin turning white as blood vessels contract, and then, due to reduced blood supply, muscles lose flexibility and functionality. That's very similar to what ice-water does to your stomach. Ice-water will constrict the blood vessels that feed the stomach muscles which then reduces the muscles' ability to provide strong peristaltic contractions. Further, ice-cold drinks effectively freeze the digestive process by causing fats to congeal (we know that liquid olive oil or butter will turn solid when refrigerated). Beginning with chewing, digestion is essentially a series of actions that liquify and break down food into smaller pieces (all the way down to the molecular level) so that nutrients can be absorbed, first through the intestinal wall and then into the cells. Freezing foods (especially fats) causes them to remain solid and clump together which is the opposite of what digestion is supposed to do.

While drinking ice-cold beverages may not result in acid reflux in all cases, if someone has a chronic issue with the upper digestive tract, discontinuing the consumption of iced drinks with meals is the most basic and prudent first course of action.

There is also a well thought out line of reasoning that acid reflux is often caused by too little stomach acid (rather than too much) which causes the partially digested food to remain in the stomach for too long. We offer detailed information about that at our store. In this case however, it seemed like more reasonable eating habits were the first thing to address.

I suggested she begin her meals with warm miso soup or mild ginger tea, chew extremely well and finish with warm herbal tea. She thanked me for the advice.

About three weeks later she returned and said that her digestive problem was essentially gone and that she had some embarrassing admissions to make. It turns out she had worked as a nurse in a doctor's office for over two decades, had worked with doctors to solve this problem for several years, and was *never* asked about the way she ate (only what she ate). Eliminating the ice-water from her meals and chewing well had completely solved her chronic digestive problems ... (**SIRS**)

Head injury:

We have seen two separate but remarkably similar stories involving head injuries, this is one of them: A woman came into our store one day looking for help, accompanied by her husband. She had been struck in the head by a line-drive at her daughter's softball practice. In the following days and weeks she had the symptoms associated with vertigo and injury – dizziness, unsteadiness, headache, visual disturbances, feelings of spinning, and sensitivity to light and sudden sounds.

She had undergone every medical test the local doctors could think of (generating a five-figure bill for her insurance company along the way) and after several weeks she still had headaches and couldn't drive or work. Based on her test results, her doctors couldn't really understand the severity of her symptoms and had no more suggestions beyond waiting, hoping, or traveling outside the area to consult with more specialists.

I suggested she see a Cranio-sacral therapist. Practitioners of Cranial-sacral therapy use their hands to gently free up restrictions in the movement of cranial bones and associated soft tissues and while stimulating the flow of the cerebrospinal fluid, which bathes all the surfaces of the brain and the spinal cord. The medical mainstream generally views Cranio-sacral therapy as complete nonsense.

After the first treatment, she felt 85% better. After the second, nearly 100% better, and after the third and final treatment she was as good as new ... **(SIRS)**

Stuttering:

While visiting friends in a different state I met a nice young family. Susan obviously loved her kids like only a mother can and was very concerned with the severe stuttering problem of her 11 year-old son, David. They had tried different behavioral, speech pattern, and breath therapies to improve his condition. Susan said that all had provided some improvement, but to my ear his stutter was still very noticeable and David appeared to be very self-conscious about it.

I had been introduced as a health food store owner. Probably because of that, Susan later pulled me aside and asked if I knew of any supplements that might help her son. I told her there were supplements he could try, but I didn't think they would provide the degree of help they were looking for.

Emotional trauma, physical injuries to the head, complications from the birthing process, and other less well defined factors, appear to be the causes of stuttering. It often resolves on its own or with the help of therapy by the end of childhood, but may stay with a person for life.

The body structures involved in speaking are controlled by the cranial nerves which exit the brain through the skull. The major structures are the mouth, tongue, throat, and vocal cords.

Also important are the diaphragm (for breath control), the trachea, and even the neck vertebrae.

Sometimes any slight misalignment of the spine, especially the vertebrae of the neck, can create tension on the fascia (connective tissue) that envelops the many structures of the throat and chest. This may interfere with proper breathing, voice production, and coordination of the many muscles (of the tongue, jaw, larynx, and diaphragm) involved in speech.

When I mention Cranio-sacral therapy to people, most have never heard of it. Cranio-sacral therapy (is based on a branch of medicine called Osteopathy) helps the body to release the tension in the connective tissue, and open up the space for all the structures contained within it.

I suggested David try a few treatments. Susan was able to find an Osteopath in their area with a good reputation for this type of work. I later found out that the results from the first treatment were dramatic and after a short series of treatments, David no longer had an obvious stutter. You gotta love it! ... **(SIRS)**

An important thing to remember about about Cranio-sacral therapy is: At this point, a large percentage of massage therapists have dabbled in, or taken a weekend workshop or two in Cranio-sacral work. For serious problems you should find one who has extensive experience and good references specifically pertaining to their Cranio-sacral abilities.

Ulcerative colitis:

About a decade ago a middle-aged woman came in to our store searching for help for her husband Larry's condition. He had suffered with doctor-diagnosed, ulcerative colitis for 20 years. Most of that time he used prescriptions to manage the inflammation and pain. For an active man with a full-time job, the accompanying weakness and weight loss during flare-ups was equally difficult to endure.

I suggested he try using a premium probiotic preparation along with a liquid herbal blend containing aloe and other herbs known for soothing and healing the stomach and intestinal linings. Within one month, Larry was able to discontinue his prescription medications. By the end of the second month he felt stronger and reestablished a healthy weight. ... **(SIRS)**

Psoriasis:

About 12 years ago, long before the recent upswing in awareness about food allergies, a 50 year-old woman came in suffering from itching and red scaly patches that had been diagnosed as Psoriasis. She had several areas on her body that had been problem spots for over decade. She had tried it all: steroid creams, vitamin A creams, extra sunlight, etc. They all provided minimal relief. She purchased some blood cleaning herbs from us – still no success.

Based on the successful treatment of Psoriasis that another customer had shared with me (pesky anecdote), I proposed that my 50 year old customer might be suffering from a food allergy or sensitivity.

I suggested that she try giving up eating the three most common food allergens, wheat, dairy products, and soy foods for a few weeks and see how her Psoriasis responded. She went on the elimination diet and her Psoriasis improved dramatically. When she began to add back the foods one at a time, it became clear that her body and wheat did not get along well at all. In fact when she reintroduced wheat back into her diet she experienced severe headaches on days when she ate wheat more than once, and the Psoriasis returned.

The next (and final) time she eliminated all gluten containing products for several months. Her headaches vanished and while she ended up with minor scars on the two of the Psoriasis affected spots, the redness, itching, and flaking were gone for good ... **(SIRS)**

A decade of coughing:

About ten years ago (again, before the medical mainstream began taking food allergies seriously), a woman appearing to be in her early to mid seventies came in complaining of a chronic cough. "How chronic is it?" I asked. She said she coughed every day for nearly a decade. She explained that she had gone to several highly regarded university medical centers in California before moving to Oregon and none provided suggestions that led to long-lasting relief without drugs.

As I often do whenever people have upper respiratory health challenges, I suggested that she might want to give up dairy foods. We spoke about food allergies and she decided to try eliminating dairy foods and wheat from her diet. After 10 years of chronic coughing, about **three** days after eliminating dairy and wheat, her cough was gone for good ... **(SIRS)**

At one time, my brother and I suffered from severe seasonal allergies. By eliminating dairy foods from our diets, we both experienced, first-hand, an immediate and unmistakable positive impact on our health. I currently live in agriculturally fertile region that is known for having high pollen counts and presenting many challenges for people with seasonal allergies. As long as I follow a dairy-free diet, I experience virtually no allergy symptoms.

Over the years I have encouraged hundreds of people who have ongoing respiratory challenges to try eliminating dairy products from their diets. Hearing feedback of life-changing health improvement stories from many of them later makes it 100% clear to me that many people experience far better health when following a dairy-free diet. Issues like sinus pressure and/or frequent sinus infections, frequent earaches and/or infections, chronic coughing, wheezing, shortness of breath, and even itchy, watery eyes are often completely "cured" by removing dairy foods from their diets.

Recently, many people are also discovering that sensitivity to gluten (the elastic, chewy protein found in wheat and some other grains) can trigger inflammatory response in their bodies that can constrict airways, contributing to many of the same respiratory difficulties mentioned in the prior paragraph. Eliminating gluten containing foods often completely "cures" those problems as well.

Combined with my personal experience, the sheer number of respiratory-health success stories I've heard from people who have eliminated one or both of those categories of foods (dairy and gluten) makes it impossible for me to ignore the value of trying these simple dietary adjustments before employing a more intrusive approach.

If you suffer from respiratory challenges and the first remedies your doctor recommends to treat those challenges include prescription medications or synthetic over the counter allergy and

cold medications, *rather than* advising you to explore dietary adjustments, it may be time to fire him and find a doctor with more experience or a broader knowledge base.

Simple hydrotherapy assists bone healing:

About two years ago an elderly woman came into our store wearing a removable plastic cast (walking boot) on her foot. She had broken her fifth metatarsal about three years earlier. She was taking an excellent calcium supplement but for some reason the bone wasn't healing properly. Her mobility was being greatly affected and unfortunately she had become quite sedentary. Her foot was often cold. Her doctor had considered surgery but in this case, the risks of anesthesia needed to be considered carefully.

Good nutrition is an important part of healing anything but it should be remembered that the nutrients need to **reach** the damaged tissue. That is the job of the blood and circulatory system. In this person's case she was getting very little physical exercise. Combined with her advanced age, this was causing her circulation to be far less than ideal. Stimulating blood flow to her foot through manual massage was painful for her.

To increase circulation in her foot for the purpose of getting more nutrients to the damaged area, I suggested she try using alternating hot and cold foot baths twice a day – soaking her foot in hot water for about three minutes until the skin was red and then running cold water over it for about a minute – and repeating the process three times ending with the hot soak. It should be noted that if there appears to be inflammation and/or swelling present (especially likely with recent injuries) it would be best to end with the cold water.

She did this hot, cold, hot regimen faithfully for about four months, at which time her surprised podiatrist declared her foot healed and she was able to shed the protective boot ... (SIRS)

Tooth pain that dentists couldn't fix:

A woman came in with her 8-year-old son. He was experiencing tooth pain (in the same tooth every night) after dinner nearly every night. She said that two different dentists could not identify any cause for the pain. I recommended she take her son to visit a local chiropractor who had an especially good reputation for having a broad knowledge base.

The chiropractor successfully treated the boy's tooth pain by focusing on the muscles that control the temporomandibular (jaw) joint. He accessed the muscles by reaching inside the boy's mouth and massaging specific areas, released tension and re-aligned the joint. One visit solved the problem ... **(SIRS)**

Earning The "Hippocrates Seal Of Approval"

That these, outside-the-mainstream-medical-box, methods are often effective is fantastic news for those of us who wish to use alternative strategies to stay well. Going further, a big part of the intrinsic beauty of the health success stories in this chapter is that even if these methods had not worked they would have caused *no harm* and were very low cost. Hippocrates would certainly approve.

A *very* important point to remember is that all health practitioners are not equally proficient. In every specialty there are excellent, good, and mediocre practitioners. You owe it to yourself to try to find the very best in your geographic area. I was once looking for a massage therapist. My favorite chiropractor and favorite acupuncturist both recommended the same person. I took that as an excellent sign and ultimately was very pleased with her skill and professionalism. I would avoid choosing a health practitioner solely by price or by how pretty their ad or website is. Ask friends, relatives, other healthcare practitioners, or other people you trust, for a recommendation. Whom you allow to work on your body is a significant decision.

By being proactive and working together sharing accurate information, we can all help chart the course of our Wellness Uprising!

Recommended Resource Guide

I highly recommend all of the following books and resources for a more in-depth understanding of many of the subjects contained in this book.

Rodale Institute – the preeminent organic farming experts since 1947. Their website offers an incredible amount of awe-inspiring information – http://rodaleinstitute.org/

Healing With Whole Foods by Paul Pitchford
A comprehensive guide to the theory and healing power of whole foods and herbs within the context of Chinese medicine theory.

Spontaneous Healing and **8 Weeks To Optimum Health** by Dr. Andrew Weil
How to discover and embrace your body's natural ability to maintain and heal itself. Philosophy, facts, practical advice, and fascinating case studies.

Encyclopedia of Natural Medicine by Dr. Michael Murray
The most comprehensive reference book of its kind (1200 pages), but still very user friendly and easy to understand. If you were to purchase only one book on natural healthcare, this should be it.

How to Raise a Healthy Child in Spite of Your Doctor by Robert S. Mendelsohn MD
Despite being written 30 years ago, this book is in many ways is still way ahead of its time. Renowned pediatrician Dr. Robert Mendelsohn reaffirms that parents can and should be the ultimate authorities for their children's health.

The Life Bridge by Paul Shulick and Thomas Newmark
Short and simple yet profound book about the importance to human health of beneficial bacteria working on many levels.

The Art of Fermentation by Sandor Ellix Katz
A truly comprehensive book about the subject of naturally fermented foods – philosophy as well as practical instruction is included – a unique and indispensable resource.

The National Vaccine Information Center (NVIC), http://www.nvic.org/
The name of their group says it all. I view them as a trustworthy resource and donate a modest sum to their cause annually.

Dr. Mercola's Vaccine Website http://vaccines.mercola.com/
Dr. Mercola is one of the prolific forces in the United States for disseminating truthful information about virtually all aspects of natural healthcare.

For more information, please contact the author directly:
Email: RobertPell9@gmail.com
Phone: 877.656.1634

Made in the USA
San Bernardino, CA
19 October 2014